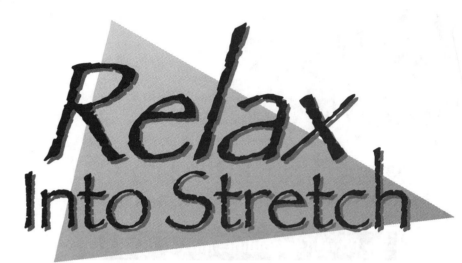

Relax Into Stretch

Instant Flexibility through Mastering Muscle Tension

By Pavel Tsatsouline, Master of Sports

I have trained Soviet commandos to DO SPLITS IN THREE TO SIX MONTHS—whether they liked it, or not.   Now that I have turned into a capitalist running dog, I will teach you too.   When I'm done with you, you'll have the flexibility of a mutant. Or else.

—Pavel Tsatsouline, Master of Sports

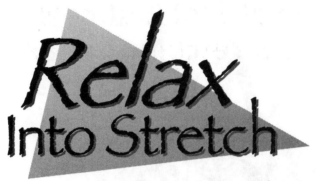

Relax Into Stretch

Instant Flexibility through Mastering Muscle Tension

By Pavel Tsatsouline, Master of Sports

Published in the United States by:
Dragon Door Publications, Inc
P.O. Box 4381, St. Paul, MN 55104
Tel: (651) 487-2180 • Fax: (651) 487-3954
Credit card orders: 1-800-899-5111
Email: dragondoor@aol.com • Website: www.dragondoor.com

ISBN: 0-938045-28-8

Book design, Illustrations and cover by Derek Brigham
Website http//www.dbrigham.com
Tel/Fax: (612) 827-3431 • Email: dbrigham@visi.com
Digital photography by Andrea Du Cane and
Robert Pearl Photography • Tel: (612) 617-7724

Manufactured in the United States
Second Edition: April 2002

DISCLAIMER
The author and publisher of this material are not responsible in any manner whatsoever for any injury that may occur through following the instructions contained in this material. The activities, physical and otherwise, described herein for informational purposes only, may be too strenuous or dangerous for some people and the reader(s) should consult a physician before engaging in them.

Praise for Pavel Tsatsouline's Beyond Stretching

"Pavel is the leading proponent of applied flexibility training for bodybuilding and strength athletics at work in the field today. His ideas are dynamic and fresh, he razes the sacred temples and shows the serious-minded fitness devotee another avenue of improvement. Real knowledge for real people interested in real progress."

—Marty Gallagher, Editor, Parrillo Preformance Press, health and fitness columnist, Washington Post.com. World Masters Powerlifting Champion

"The foremost authority, critic, and writer in the emerging "science of flexibility" is a Russian physiologist, Pavel Tsatsouline. His book *Beyond Stretching* is without question the definitive text on the subject. It is MUST READING for every athlete…YOU HAVE TO GET A COPY OF IT!"

—Judd Biasiotto, Ph.D., Powerlifting USA, Emmy award winner, sports psychologist and writer, Four-time Powerlifting World Record Holder

"Pavel has great ideas on flexibility and strength exercises. We agree on all aspects of flexibility."

—Bill Superfoot, Wallace, M.Sc., World Kickboxing Champion

"As an athlete, a coach, and a strength trainer who has personally done it all in the sports world from martial arts to the NFL, I have always experimented on me first when I read something as radical as *Beyond Stretching*. When I went into my first, full-to-the-floor splits in ten years, after just three weeks, I realized why this Russian was so cocky. It's because he is so damned right"

— Carter Stamm, New Orleans, LA

"Here are a book and video that present a revolutionary Russian system of stretching that's easy to do and get results fast.

I wrote in my review of Pavel Tsatsouline's book *Power to the People!: Russian Strength Training Secrets for Every American* that Pavel's methods get results while violating many of the "truths" that have been held as sacred for so long in the world of strength development.

In *Beyond Stretching: Russian Flexibility Breakthroughs*, he again offers result-producing methods, this time for increasing flexibility, while again violating what has been held as truths ever since you were in grade school gym class.
Pavel's writing style is no nonsense, efficient and quite often funny. If you are looking to be coddled, you won't get it from him. He tells you when something is tough and then he tells you to do it any way. The beauty of it is when you do what he says, you will begin seeing progress in a couple of weeks.

I have been training in the martial arts for nearly 36 years and, as such, stretching exercises have been part of my regular routine. As a result, I'm more flexible than the average guy. After reading this book and viewing the video, I tried four of Pavel's exercises. Three weeks later, my flexibility had improved by about 20 percent. At this rate, I figure I'll be able to scratch my head with my big toe in a couple more months.
—Loren W. Christensen, author of The Fighter's Fact Book, Fighting Power and Speed Training

"This is the only really interesting book on stretching I've encountered.
Pavel's ideas are radical, but sensible if you think them through and apply them carefully.

His joint mobility drills alone are worth the price. Much of this book is geared towards the elite athlete who is already far along the learning curve. Nevertheless, as a reasonably in shape middle-aged guy with increasingly creaky joints, I found this book to be an invaluable resource. Buy the book and the video. You'll get your money's worth."
—Kenneth W. Robinson

"Pavel's stretching protocol should be considered the first, last, and only choice for athletes, full-contact fighters, and sedentary folks alike for achieving maximum results in minimal time. This system actually teaches you how to reset the neuro-muscular control of your muscles! No kidding, by following the specialized methods in this book, even an untrained, middle aged man can achieve FULL SPLITS in less than half a year... fighters will learn specialized kicking drills and "dynamic flexibility" drills that greatly improve the velocity and destructive power of your kicks while at the same time protecting the knee ligaments from injury—even if you miss a full-power kick!

I am shocked and amazed at the quality of the results that his training methods have produced for me. And in so little time! There is something here for everyone, and I give this book (and all Pavel's books) my highest recommendation. Truly, a masterpiece that belongs in every athlete's collection."
—Sean Williams, Long Beach, NY

"This book is well written (even a little funny!) and has some great info about stretching. It dispels a lot of classic stretching myths and gives some good solid approaches to achieving better flexibility. It's helping me become more flexible a lot faster than I was progressing using the "classical" approach. It's a must for martial artists! Check it out."
— Chris Pellitteri, Upland, CA

"Lots of useful information on improving flexibility and avoiding injury. I like Pavel's no-nonsense writing style. I got immediate benefits from reading it!"
— Bill Gillis, Boston, MA

To Mom

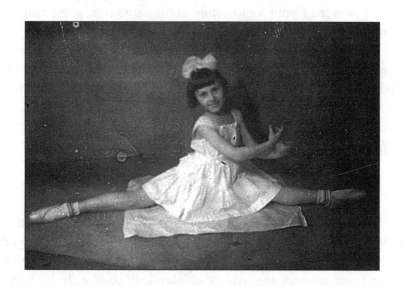

Foreword

Dear Comrade:

The readers of my earlier work *Beyond Stretching* have reported great gains in their flexibility. They also noted that some of the exercises were not very user-friendly and were difficult to organize into a personal program.

Not any more.

In the three years since the release of *Beyond Stretching* I have given many flexibility seminars to a variety of groups, ranging from mere mortals to elite martial artists and SWAT officers. However, I did not just teach, I also learned from my students. I presented a large volume of material from a great variety of sources and countries. The information ranged from the latest academic research, to the intuitive discoveries of esoteric martial arts.

I watched what clicked and ruthlessly eliminated the exercises and techniques that were either difficult to learn or less than maximally effective. The result is *Relax into Stretch: Instant Flexibility through Mastering Muscle Tension*, your friendly new shortcut to having the flexibility of a mutant.

—*Pavel Tsatsouline, Master of Sports*
January 2001, Santa Monica, California

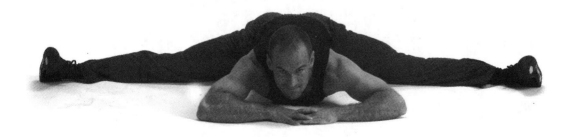

Table of Contents

The *Relax into Stretch* drills— a quick reference   **Page 47**

How much flexibility do you really need?   **Page 93**

Why excessive flexibility can be detrimental to athletic performance • why old school strongmen instinctively avoided stretching • what stretches powerlifters and weightlifters do and don't need • warning examples from sprinting, boxing and kickboxing.

When flexibility is hard to come by, build strength   **Page 96**

Plateau-busting strategies for the chronically inflexible • *high total time under tension.*

Two more plateau busting strategies from the iron world   **Page 97**

Popenko's flexibility data • the reminiscence effect • the dynamic stereotype • How to exceed your old limits with the stepwise progression.

Advanced Russian Drills for Extreme Flexibility— A Quick Reference   **Page 99**

Relax into Stretch delivers instant flexibility!   **Page 138**

Stretching is <u>NOT</u> the best way to become flexible!

Honest ignorance is better than simulated understanding.

—Judd Biasiotto, Ph.D.,
sports scientist, world champion powerlifter

Stretching in America is a cult. Every fitness-junkie guru preaches flexibility. They growl, they drool and they promise hell to the infidels who don't or won't stretch. Yet the stretching methods they offer are at best laughable, at worst dangerous.

Americans lose flexibility as they grow older because they are used to relying on the elasticity of their tissues. A lifetime of activity builds up microtrauma in our muscles, tendons and fascia. When it heals, a scar is formed. It pulls the wound together, making the muscle shorter. Some American doctors believe that relaxed stretching after exercise can prevent the muscle from healing at a shorter length. That point of view gives credibility to some sick stretching methods.

I heard that sumo wrestlers used to assume their deepest split position, then have their sensei jump on their thighs to rip the tissues and bring the big boy down to a full split. In a few weeks or months the ground meat supposedly healed at a new length and splits were no longer a problem. I do not know if someone was pulling my leg with this story, but I do know an aerobic instructor who purposefully tears her hamstrings by overstretching them, then spends hours in that position to insure that the muscles will heal at a new, greater, length. Sick—very sick.

Even if you could prevent the muscle from shortening—and that is questionable—a stiffening of the tendons and ligaments is certain. "There isn't an exercise that can prevent the aging of connective tissues. It's as certain as radioactive decay," quipped Academician Nikolay Amosov from the former USSR.

Ligaments and tendons are made of collagen, which gives them strength, and elastin, which, as its name implies, provides elasticity. As you age, the elastin/collagen ratio changes in favor of collagen, or scar tissue. If you relied on tissue elasticity for flexibility, you can kiss your flexibility good-bye. And if you put up a fight and try to literally stretch yourself, change the mechanical properties of your muscles, tendons and ligaments, your desperate attempts will bring more injuries than flexibility.

Why traditional stretching failed you, or 'garbage in, garbage out'

The traditional Western approach to flexibility has failed because it started with the assumption that muscles and connective tissues need to be physically stretched. Other myths snowball from there. Hackers have a saying, "Garbage in, garbage out." If the premise is false, all the conclusions will be wrong, no matter how sterling is the logic leading up to them.

Let it sink in: the premise that you need to stretch if you want to be flexible is wrong.

Ugh? How can it be?

Try this test. Can you extend one leg to the side at a ninety-degree angle?

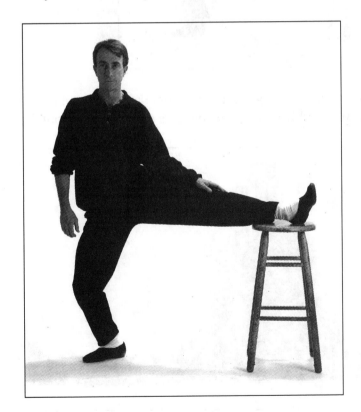

Your leg that is up on the table is now in the position for a side split. Now do it with the other leg:

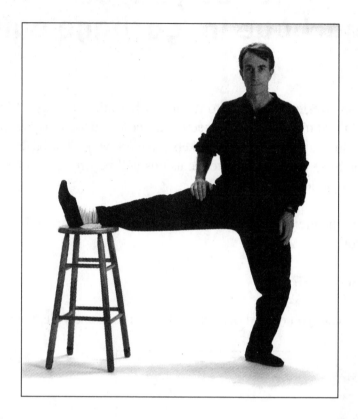

So, what stops you from spreading both legs at the same time and doing what Americans call 'the Russian split' and Russian ballet dancers call 'the dead split'?

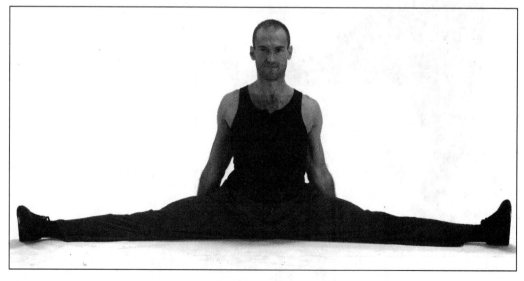

No chuckles of 'simulated understanding', please, Comrade!

No, it has nothing to do with your 'short muscles'.

Listen to this: **no muscles run from one leg to the other. No tendons, no ligaments, nothing but skin.** Like the wheels on your Land Rover, your legs boast independent suspension. That means you should be able to bring the other leg out at the same angle and do a split without stretching a thing.

So why can't you?

Fear. Tension. The muscles tighten up and resist lengthening. Russian scientists call it *antagonist passive insufficiency*.

Based on your previous experiences— sitting all day or performing monotonous labor, or exercising incorrectly—your nervous system has picked the favorite length for every one of your muscles and prefers to keep it that way. Whenever you reach too far compared to this standard, the *stretch reflex* kicks in and reins your muscles in.

If you try something really aggressive that you have never done before—for instance splits—the stretch reflex panics and stiffens up your muscles with all its might.

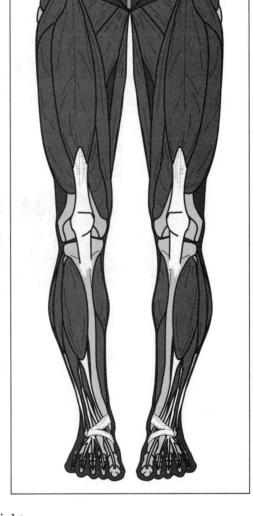

Comrade, it is not short muscles and connective tissues that make you tight; it is your nervous system, 'the muscle software' that refuses to let your muscles to slide out to their true full length! A muscle with pre-Depression connective tissues and more scars than a prize fighter is still long enough to display as much flexibility as allowed by its associated joints. Master the muscular tension—and you will be as flexible as you want to be, at any age.

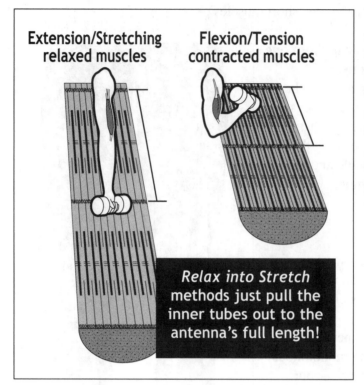

Extension/Stretching
relaxed muscles

Flexion/Tension
contracted muscles

Relax into Stretch
methods just pull the
inner tubes out to the
antenna's full length!

If you compare your muscle to a telescopic antenna, conventional stretching mangles the outer tube in a vain attempt to elongate it. In contrast, *Relax into Stretch* methods just pull the inner tubes out to the antenna's full length!

Reclaim the buoyant flexibility of your youth—and more

In order to get super flexible you must do three things.

1) Trick your muscles into relaxation with various natural reflexes.

A reflex is your body's automatic response to some stimulus. For example, the stretch reflex that contracts your muscles in response to stretching is not voluntary, 'it just happens'. The human organism sports many such reflexes that make your life easier by responding to various standard situations without calling the HQ, or your brain, for every stupid thing. To give you another example, blinking in response to fast movement near your face is a reflex that protects your eyes. You get the idea.

The reflexes form a hierarchy where some of them may override others because they have more 'stripes'. *Relax into Stretch* teaches you how to inhibit the stretch reflex with other reflexes that are higher up in the food chain.

2) Convince your nervous system that the new range of motion is safe.

The first step has taken you there half way. Once your muscles have been duped into relaxing against their will, they will face the music. Your stretch reflex will think, "Hey, the muscle is longer but it hasn't ripped in half! This isn't as bad as I thought."

Now make sure to progress at a very conservative pace. Pay constant attention to a sense of safety in your stretching, to keep your nervous system relaxed and happy. If you do not feel safe in some precarious position, your muscles will refuse to relax.

Building strength in the stretched position will also go a long way towards confidently releasing your muscles into a super stretch.

3) Create the new 'habitual' muscle length.

There are two ways to create a new habit: extensive and intensive.

A good example of extensive learning is memorizing your boss's phone number after you have dialed it a hundred times. Contrast that with the instant filing away of the phone number of a traffic-stopping lady you have just met. It sure worked for me when I met my future wife.

Applied to stretching, extensive learning refers to holding the final stretched out position for as long as you can stand it. Repetition will reset the standard of length. The intensive method calls for brief but intense stimulation with powerful techniques that involve intense muscular contraction. To get the best effect, both extensive and intensive methods are employed.

Once you do all of the above—full splits are yours!

Waiting out the Tension—
relaxed stretching as it should be

The most obvious way to control muscular tension is … well, just relax.

Get in a comfortably stretched position and stay in it until your muscles relax. It usually takes a couple of minutes—although timing yourself is a decidedly bad idea. The relaxation time will vary greatly depending on your training level, fatigue, stress, the given muscle group, and many other variables. Just listen to your body.

The technique of *Waiting out the Tension* works well only in select lower body stretches that are comfortable enough to stay in for a long time. For instance, the Leg Straddle is a winner and the Good Morning is not.

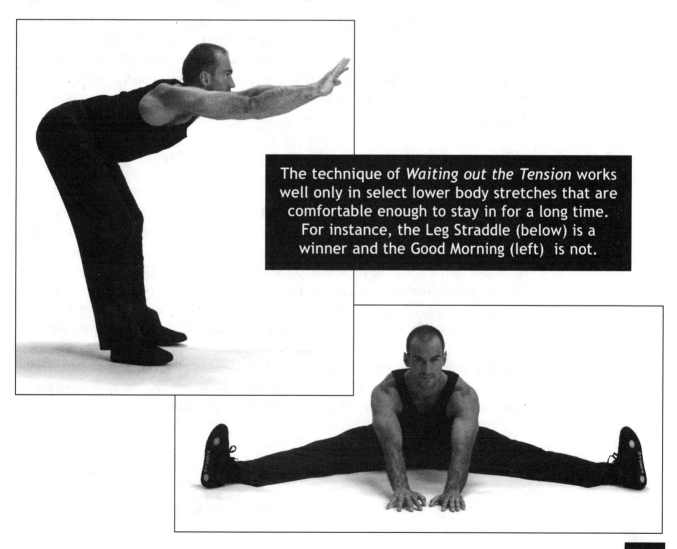

The technique of *Waiting out the Tension* works well only in select lower body stretches that are comfortable enough to stay in for a long time. For instance, the Leg Straddle (below) is a winner and the Good Morning (left) is not.

Once the muscle has relaxed, increase the stretch. Your muscles will tighten up again. One more time, wait the tension out. Breathe deep, easy, and slow. Repeat until you are close to getting spasms.

If you paid attention, you have understood that what has been described is not the literal stretching of a relaxed muscle, but rather a patient **waiting for the muscle to relax and picking up the slack.**

Your reflexes, like everything else in your body, get tired.

When the doctor taps your quad tendon with a hammer, your leg kicks out and the muscle gets stretched. If the doctor persisted at whacking you under your kneecap, your kicks would get progressively weaker and weaker until the hammer could not get a rise out of you at all. By the same token, if your muscles tighten up once you have assumed a stretched position, you can wait the stretch reflex out.

This involuntary neural mechanism is what makes your muscles resist the stretch. If you stay down long enough, usually a couple of minutes, the stretch reflex will get tired of firing up your muscles, allowing them to finally relax. Now it is time to carefully increase the range of motion until the muscles start resisting, and repeat the process… You may massage the stretched muscles and/or gently 'twitch' them once in a while to help the relaxation process and ease the discomfort.

If you would like to know why these maneuvers help, read my book *Fast & Loose!: Russian Champions' Dynamic Relaxation Secrets.*

While many Russians and Orientals have been successful with *Waiting out the Tension,* I believe that Americans are generally not patient enough to stretch in this manner. No offense intended, just a cultural observation. You guys tend to get eager and start forcing the muscle into more stretch. The results are injuries and zero progress. Perhaps you will overcome your busy nature by following the example of world champion kickboxer Bill 'Superfoot' Wallace who stretches at night in front of the TV when he is not in a hurry and does not feel competitive.

From personal experience I can tell you that you should never, ever stretch when you are tight on time, no pun intended. Rushing through your stretches makes it impossible to relax, delivers no gains, and almost guarantees injuries.

Do not abuse relaxed stretches and stay away from them altogether when it comes to your back. Soviet sports scientist L. P. Orlov warns: "While most large joints are stabilized by muscles and the ligaments do not affect their position, in the case of the spine it is the ligaments that play the important role of maintaining the normal spinal alignment. Insufficiency of the ligamentous apparatus makes it difficult to maintain the normal spinal curve with muscle tonus and tension alone. Weakening of the ligaments unavoidably leads to deformation of the spinal column."

In other words, don't do relaxed stretches for forward flexion of your spine or toe touching.

And make sure that *Waiting out the Tension* is not the only stretching method you employ. "Flexibility must always be in a certain relationship with strength," Orlov states—and unlike *Forced Relaxation* and other specialized techniques you are about to learn, *Waiting out the Tension* does not develop strength.

Finally, if you insist on doing relaxed stretches, remember the words of a famous Russian coach who said that in sports conditioning—as in an intimate situation—trying too hard just dooms one to failure. Do not will your muscles to relax. Let it happen.

Waiting out the Tension

- Get in a comfortably stretched position and patiently stay in it for a few minutes until your muscles relax.

- Increase the stretch. Your muscles will tighten up again. One more time, wait the tension out. Breathe deep and easy. Repeat until you are close to getting spasms.

- You may massage the stretched muscles and/or gently 'twitch' them once in a while to help the relaxation process and ease the discomfort.

- The technique of *Waiting out the Tension* works well only in select stretches that are comfortable enough to stay in for a long time.

- Never use the *Waiting out the Tension* for forward spine flexion or toe touching type stretches

- **Don't** get eager and start forcing the muscle into more stretch.

- **Never** stretch when you are in a hurry

- **Don't** apply the *Waiting out the Tension* technique to your back.

A split, a fire walk, an act of faith...

Victor Popenko's 1994 book *Flexibility, Strength, Endurance,* became a bestseller among the Russian Mafia enforcers, who pride themselves on being the best-conditioned bad guys in the world. Popenko writes:

"The key to mobility is relaxation. Usually the body possesses great stretching reserves but the stretched muscle is resisting by trying to contract, and this resistance must be overcome with the psychological mindset on relaxation.

Stretching exercises must be performed slowly and carefully, with a fixation of the stretched position for a minute or so. While holding the stretch all your intentions should be on relaxation, a reduction of tension in the stretched muscles. Such mental concentration enables one to reach stunning results.

Appropriate images and pictures sometimes help the relaxation mindset. For example, imagine that your legs are the ends of a rope easily spread apart as you perform a split. Visualizing heat is very helpful. Mentally wrap the spot with most muscular tension with a hot towel in a few layers. As this hot application heats up, the muscle softens up and relaxes.

Be persistent in your desire to relax the stretched muscles. Every time you succeed, you have succeeded in stretching yourself a little further."

A suspended side split, like a fire walk, is an act of faith. This is not psychobabble, this is a fact.

There is an intimate connection between the limbic system, which governs the emotions, and the neural networks that govern muscular length and tension. Scientific studies show that fear and anxiety, as well as pain, reduce flexibility.

With that in mind, maximize the safety of your stretches—and their *perceived* safety. If it takes three chairs, a step stool, and a spotter to make you feel safe during your splits—so be it. The reasons for your fear may not be real, but it wipes out your flexibility for real just the same.

If you do not believe that you can do a wishbone, you never will. And vice versa. Confidence and yoga-like tranquility allow extreme flexibility to happen.

Although not a must, various tools for relaxing the body and the mind from sports psychology and Oriental self-improvement disciplines—such as the *Jacobson's Progressive Relaxation Technique* and *Chi Kung* meditation, will ease your ascension to the rank of superflexible mutants. The unique vibration drills of Russian champions from my book and tape *Fast & Loose!* are guaranteed to be of great help.

Another relaxation tip. Drs. Yuri Verkhoshansky and Mel Siff, renowned sports scientists and the authors of *Supertraining,* advise controlling muscular tension in the face and hands, because it reflects overall tension. Indeed, your face and your hands have a much greater nerve supply than the rest of the body—you could say that they own the controlling interest in your relaxation stock.

Relaxation Tips

- Focus your intentions on the relaxation of your muscles and mind.

- Appropriate visualizations, for example heat, help relaxation.

- Anxiety and pain reduce flexibility. Reduce them by progressing at a comfortable pace and maximizing the safety of your stretches.

- Consider taking up meditation, the *Jacobson's Progressive Relaxation Technique,* or some other relaxation technique from sports psychology and Oriental self-improvement disciplines. The vibration and passive movement drills from *Fast & Loose!* are awesome.

- Control muscular tension in the face and hands because it reflects overall tension. Literally 'wipe' the tension off your face with your palms, slowly and firmly, from top to bottom.

Proprioceptive Neuromuscular Facilitation—if you can spell it, splits ought to be a piece of cake!

A more proactive way to relax the muscle into the stretch is *proprioceptive neuromuscular facilitation,* a spelling test nightmare from the physical therapists' arsenal.

Developed by the American Dr. Henry Kabat, half a century ago, PNF works by fooling your stretch reflex. Here you are, stretched out to what your body thinks is the limit. The muscle does not seem to be able to get any tenser. Yet you make it happen by flexing it.

Everything in this world is relative. What felt maximally tense before the contraction, does not feel quite as tight in the aftermath. You eke out a little more stretch.

Put more scientifically: Contracting a muscle inhibits the stretch reflex in this muscle, via an element in your spinal cord called a *Renshaw cell.* Essentially the *Renshaw cell* tells the stretch reflex, "Hey, don't panic, man! The muscle is already contracting, no sense in overdoing it."

It has been known since Russian dog abuser Pavlov's times that neural processes are inert—they respond to stuff with some delay. They are like those dull-witted comrades whom we called 'brakes' in the Russian military.

Applied to stretching, this means that after you terminate a contraction, the stretch reflex in the given muscle will still be temporarily suppressed—and the muscle will not resist stretching much. At least for a little while. The window of opportunity is narrow: studies show that the muscle's resistance to stretch is minimal within the first second after the contraction; by the fifth second it is up to 70% of the initial tension, then it is back to square one.

To sum up the standard PNF technique, contract the stretched muscle for the specified duration, anywhere from a second to a few minutes, then relax it, and immediately—understand the difference between 'immediately' and 'rapidly' for your own good!—stretch the temporarily cooperating muscle a little further.

If you prefer a less geeky term than PNF, you may call any technique that involves pre-tensing of the stretched muscle *contract-relax stretching* or *isometric stretching*.

Isometric stretching rules!

Contract-relax stretching is documented to be at least 267% more effective than conventional relaxed stretching! In addition to fooling the stretch reflex in the manner just described, isometric stretches enhance your flexibility by making you stronger in the stretched position.

Relaxed stretching develops flexibility without strength. This is unnatural. Normally your body does not allow a range of motion it cannot control. A graphic illustration of this is a medical condition known as the 'frozen shoulder'. If, after an injury, you do not use your shoulder for a long time, it will lose much of its range of motion. Under anesthesia though, the surgeon can turn the shoulder through three hundred sixty degrees without trouble.

When the patient wakes up and his muscles start working, the shoulder freezes again. The nervous system knows that the muscles are not strong enough to control the full range motion and will not let the shoulder's owner have it. Without proper rehab the problem keeps feeding on itself. Physical therapists know that muscles habitually kept in a shortened position lose their strength in the stretched position. Before you know it, the weakness-inflexibility vicious circle turns you into a piece of furniture!

The same situation, albeit less extreme, repeats itself with every Joe or Jane when they work out improperly—or are simply inathletic. Your muscles keep losing their strength in the lengthened position—if they ever had it to start with—because your lifestyle always keeps them shortened. Physical therapists call this problem 'tight weakness'. As strength goes south, so does flexibility. The muscles become even shorter which makes them even weaker which makes them even shorter… ad nauseam.

And vice versa.   When you become stronger in the extreme range of motion through contract-relax stretching, you send the message to your body that you will not be stuck in that position because you now have the strength to recover from it. Your muscles do not undergo a reflexive contraction since your nervous system perceives the stretch as safe. Your flexibility increases.

The obvious way to develop extreme range strength is by lifting weights but it is not always practical. You get stronger primarily at the angles where you train. If you can do full one hundred eighty-degree splits, it is worthless to use a health club adductor/abductor machine limited to one hundred and twenty degrees.

Isometrics is more practical than weights. You are probably familiar with isometric strength training. It was very popular in the fifties and sixties. You had to push against things that didn't budge, like walls, doorways, or trucks. Your muscles contracted but no movement took place. Isometrics is a very powerful tool for strength development, despite being out of favor and receiving much unjust criticism in the last few decades.

John Ziegler, M.D., one of the pioneers of isometric strength training, explained how it works: "…the way you improve is by lifting weights, the heaviest possible. What's the heaviest weight you can lift?—One you can't lift!"

To develop strength-flexibility with isometrics, stretch as far as you can, then flex the stretched muscle. Sounds just like isometric stretching, doesn't it?

Extreme flexibility through *Contrast Breathing*

The effectiveness of conventional PNF can be dramatically increased through proper breathing. Take a lesson from Chi Kung, Tai Chi and Yoga. Masters of these Oriental disciplines put heavy emphasis on breathing exercises that leads to remarkable mastery of the body and mind. Here is why.

Your nervous system is subdivided into *voluntary*, which is in charge of things like lifting your arm or chewing your cheeseburger, and *autonomic*, which quietly runs things that are none of your business, like digesting that cheeseburger.

Breathing is the only function you can control both consciously and unconsciously because it is regulated by both branches of the nervous system through two independent sets of nerves. By controlling your breathing, you can control some of your body's functions that were never meant to be controlled voluntarily, like your heart rate.

Note how forcing yourself to 'take a deep breath' when you freak out helps to calm you down. Because deep, relaxed breathing is incompatible with a stressed out mind, your body adjusts its physiology to your breathing via a feedback loop! Quoting Harvard M. D. and alternative medicine guru Andrew Weil, "Breathing is the bridge between mind and body, the connection between consciousness and unconsciousness."

Here is how you can breathe your way to greater flexibility. Get in the position of a comfortable stretch, placing some weight on the muscles you are stretching.

Inhale maximally and tighten up your entire body, especially the target muscles.

The deepest relaxation can only be achieved in contrast to great tension—the yin and yang of stretching, so to say. Or, if you prefer the Marxist terminology, 'the unity and antagonism of the polarities'.

Think of your body as a fist. Literally making a fist will help. Pay attention not to decrease the amount of stretch when you are tightening up!

Hold your breath—and tension—for a second or so, then suddenly let it all out with a sigh of relief. Let your jaw and shoulders go limp with the rest of your body. Let your fists and face play dead. Turn your whole body into what Soviet psychologist Dr. Vladimir Levi called 'a mentally relaxed fist'.

Visualize transforming from a tight spring into a limp noodle in a blink of an eye. A burst balloon is another useful analogy. Or try this vivid description of the tension/release sequence by Dr. Judd Biasiotto:

"You must relax instantly. To better illustrate what it would feel like to "turn off" as you have been instructed, picture yourself exerting all your strength in an effort to push a large boulder off a sheer cliff. When suddenly the boulder goes over the edge, there is no active resistance to your pushing and all your straining suddenly ceases. It is that feeling, that nothingness after the boulder drops, that you are striving to obtain when you "turn off your source of power."

At this point the stretch will increase, as the involved body parts will drop down when the tension is released. To make your stretches safer, don't let the body parts drop more than an inch or so at a time. Keep repeating the drill until you can no longer increase your range of motion.

Because you are taking deep breaths, you are apt to hyperventilate. Don't. In addition to making you dizzy, washing too much carbon dioxide out of your system, by breathing too much, will excite your nervous system. While powerlifters like to take advantage of this phenomenon when psyching up for a heavy attempt, it will make it harder for you to relax. A simple way to handle the problem is to postpone the inhalation by a couple of seconds following each exhalation: hold your 'no-breath'.

Contrast Breathing is by far the easiest and least uncomfortable variation of contract-relax stretching. Obviously, if it gets you to your goals, *Contrast Breathing* is the approach of choice. If not—read on!

Contrast Breathing

- Inhale maximally and tighten up your entire body, especially the muscles you are about to stretch. Think of your body as a fist. Literally making a fist will help.

- Pay attention not to decrease the amount of stretch when you are tightening up!

- Hold your breath—and tension—for a second or so, then suddenly let it all out with a sigh of relief. Let your jaw and shoulders go limp with the rest of your body. Let your fists and face play dead. Turn your whole body into 'a mentally relaxed fist'.

- The stretch will increase as the involved body parts drop down when the tension is released. **Don't** let them drop more than an inch or so at a time, to make your stretches safer.

- With the exception of the forward bending backstretches, you may stay in the relaxed position for awhile before the next contraction.

- Keep repeating the sequence until you can no longer increase your range of motion.

- Don't hyperventilate, or take in too much air. Compensate for deep breaths by breathing less frequently; hold the 'no-breath' for a couple of seconds following each exhalation.

- You can expand your understanding of the pneumo-muscular reflex and the effect of breathing on muscle tension by reading *Power to the People!: Russian Strength Secrets for Every American.*

Forced Relaxation—the Russian spirit of stretching

Although the primitive standard PNF protocol does improve flexibility better than conventional relaxed stretching—and builds some strength in the process—there are tricks of the trade that turn the contract-relax approach into a thermonuclear stretching weapon!

Take *'Forced Relaxation'*, an oxymoronic technique which should have been invented by the Russian military. Get into the stretch, then contract the specified muscles with one to two thirds of your maximum effort. Hold steady, unwavering tension—it is extremely important! If you were holding a real weight with the target muscle, the weight would stay put rather than bob up and down.

Don't hold your breath. Breathe, but breathe shallow. Deep breathing will wave the tension in the stretched muscle up and down with every breath, something we are trying to avoid.

Hold the tension until it becomes unbearable, then release it with a sigh of relief—don't let the breath get 'caught' in your chest, as is common for a very stressed out person, let go! —and immediately increase the stretch.

If you have the mental fortitude, keep the tension until your muscles start quivering and finally collapse in exhaustion, unable to contract any longer! This is the essence of *Forced Relaxation*. Aptly named, isn't it? As we used to say in the Soviet Special Forces, "If you don't know how—we'll teach you, if you don't want to—we'll make you."

How long will you have to hold? It is hard to tell. Fifteen seconds, thirty seconds, a minute, even more. It depends on a whole lot of variables: the intensity of the contraction, your pain tolerance, and the muscle fiber type.

Drs. Verkhoshansky and Siff point out in *Supertraining* that "…prolonged muscle contraction would tend to be more easily maintained in slow postural (tonic) than in fast (phasic) muscles. Consequently, stretching procedures would have to be applied for longer periods on slow muscles to significantly enhance their flexibility."

No, you do not need a biopsy to determine the fast/slow fiber composition of your various muscles. Trial and error will do. Over a period of time you will find your sweet spot. For instance, you may observe that your hamstrings relax just fine after ten second contractions—while your hip flexors need a solid minute of tension before they are forced into exhaustion.

Forced Relaxation

- Stretch as far as comfortably possible and contract the muscles you are about to stretch with one to two thirds of your maximum effort.

- Tension should increase gradually and reach its peak by the third or fourth second. **Don't** contract the stretched muscles explosively!

- Hold steady, unwavering tension. If you were holding a real weight with the target muscle, the weight would stay put rather than bob up and down.

- **Don't** hold your breath, breathe shallow.

- Hold the tension until it becomes unbearable, then release it with a sigh of relief—**don't** let the breath get 'caught' in your chest as is common for a very stressed out person; let go! —and immediately increase the stretch.

- Understand that 'immediately' means 'without delay' rather than 'with quick movement'!

- The duration of the contraction may vary from five seconds to five minutes. Find your sweet spot through trial and error. Start with thirty to sixty second contractions.

- If you have the mental fortitude, keep the tension until your muscles start quivering and finally collapse in exhaustion, unable to contract any longer.

- Use your head (duh!)

The final frontier: why *Clasp Knife* stretches will work when everything else fails

I feel your pain, my fellow Americans.
—Bill Clinton

A kickboxer who had practiced mainstream PNF diligently for years came to me as the last resort. He was only three inches off the ground in the side split, yet never got any deeper. 'Experts' had told him it was not meant to be, he was not built for splits and too old. With the variation of isometric stretching described in this chapter, I put him in a full Russian split in ten minutes, screams notwithstanding.

This powerful variation of isometric stretching, 'the Clasp Knife' method, does not bother tricking the stretch reflex; it aggressively cancels it out!

The *Clasp Knife* takes advantage of nasty muscle software called the *inverse stretch reflex*. It does not take an Einstein to figure out that if the stretch reflex makes the muscles contract, its counterpart makes them relax. You have run across the inverse stretch reflex's dirty work when you got whipped in arm wrestling. One moment your biceps is super tense—the next it turns to jello. Some neuroscientists and physical therapists liken this process to a jackknife's blade suddenly giving way—hence 'Clasp Knife' stretching.

Where *Forced Relaxation* exhausted your muscles into submission, the *Clasp Knife* takes them by storm.

The inverse stretch reflex is the last line of defense against injuries. It takes over where the stretch reflex leaves off. As the muscle is fighting an overwhelming force it gets very tense. The tension sensors—the *III and IV afferent free nerve endings* and the *Golgi tendon organs*—send a 'Relax!' command to their muscle, to prevent it from ripping its tendons off their attachments.

Now, stop mumbling, "Is it safe, is it safe?" You sound like the Nazi dentist from *The Marathon Man*. The good news is that the shutdown threshold is set up very conservatively. Much more force is needed for the tissue to rupture than it takes to make your biceps give out; a tendon is usually two to three times stronger than its muscle!

Although it feels weird and scary—your overpowered muscles start shaking and finally give out against overwhelming resistance—the inverse stretch reflex overrides the stretch reflex and promotes a very deep relaxation of the tortured muscle.

What you get is a mega-stretching tool—for those with the heart to handle it.

The Clasp Knife—or 'shutdown threshold isometrics' as it was referred to it in my earlier book—trigger the inverse stretch reflex to relax a muscle so you can then stretch it. The half-hearted contractions practiced by most physical therapists are way too wimpy to trigger the clasp knife effect.

Eastern European experts state that the Golgi tendon organs with the highest threshold cause the greatest relaxation. That means muscle tension must be extremely high. You must put weight on the stretched muscles and contract them to the hilt. It is very painful—scream your heart out!

East German specialists Drs. J. Hartmann and H. Tunnemann recommended seven second long powerful contractions alternated with six second relaxations when one aims to set off the Golgi tendon reflex. Russian scientist Dr. Leonid Matveyev advises five to six second long contractions and emphasizes that tension should increase gradually and reach its peak by the third or fourth second. A rapid buildup of tension in a stretch may result in an injury.

"Have the strength to force the moment to its crisis." These words by Thomas Stearns Eliot could be the motto of this super stretching technique.

The Clasp Knife

- Stretch as far as comfortably possible and contract the muscles you are about to stretch with a near maximum effort.
- Tension should increase gradually and reach its peak by the third or fourth second. **Don't** contract the stretched muscles explosively!
- **Don't** hold your breath, breathe shallow during the contraction.
- Hold steady high tension for five to seven seconds or so until your overpowered muscles start shaking and finally give out. If the muscles do not collapse—it may take some practice—release the tension voluntarily.
- Let out a sigh of relief identical to the one used in *Contrast Breathing* as you release the tension.
- Increase the stretch, carefully but without delay.
- Stay relaxed for five to seven seconds and repeat the sequence.
- Exercise good judgement.

Why you should not stretch your ligaments—and how you can tell if you are

I repeat, stretching the ligaments is unnecessary even for the performance of the most advanced gymnastic or martial arts skills! Your muscles have plenty of length to allow you to do splits, you just have to learn how to relax them.

Stay away from this kind of stretch

You can accomplish the splits—even the suspended wishbone—by reeducating the nervous system. But some Yoga asanas—the goraksha asana, the sakthi chalini, the khanda peeda asana, the gomukhasana to name a few—can only be performed by stretching the ligaments. The same goes for some popular Western stretches, including the notorious hurdler's stretch. Stay the hell away from them! They offer no athletic benefits whatsoever—at least not for our species.

Ligaments hold your joints together. They do not stretch well, except in children. Stretch a ligament by only six percent and it will tear. Even if you manage to stretch it without ripping it, do not consider yourself lucky. A ligament that has been subjected to excessive stretching undergoes microtears, gets scarred up, elongated, and weakened: a so-called plastic deformity. A stretched ligament means a loose and unstable joint just waiting for a severe injury. Or osteoarthritis; joint hypermobility leads to degenerative changes in the cartilage padding the joint.

How can you tell if you are stretching a ligament?

If you feel discomfort or pain in the joint, you are probably doing it. For example, your hamstrings meet their tendons a few inches above your knees. If you feel a pull in the back of your knee during a hamstring stretch, obviously you are loading the ligaments and joint capsules rather than stretching your hammies. The solution is to bend the knee slightly to unload the ligaments and refocus the stretch on the area between your glutes and a hand's width above your knees.

The normal sensations during proper flexibility training are muscle tension—which may be painful.

Stretching when injured

Rehabilitation is not my area of expertise. Over the years I have learned to talk only about the things that I know something about, so I'll keep it brief. I will also limit my reflected rehab advice to minor muscle tears—everything else is your doctor's problem.

In one sentence, RICE it, then stretch it. I will not babble about RICE—Rest, Ice, Compression and Elevation—because everybody else does. On to stretching.

Do it. ASAP, certainly within 24 hours. When a muscle tears, so do blood vessels. Internal bleeding causes the muscle to contract, a typical reaction to any foreign matter.

When a muscle gets injured, it retreats into spasm—just in case. This creates a couple of problems. First, healing takes forever. Hypertonicity restricts circulation. This is a useful feature immediately after the injury, to keep the swelling down, but counterproductive after a day or two.

Second, as a result of limited blood supply and inactivity, the muscle atrophies. And third, flexibility is lost. When a muscle spends much time in a shortened position, the stretch reflex becomes overly sensitive. A shorter muscle length and excessive tonus become the norm.

A weaker and tighter muscle will lead to more problems down the line. It is likely to get reinjured, and so are other, healthy, muscles, as a result of imbalance or compensation.

So stretch the damn thing! Find whatever hurts the most and do it, stopping just short of PAIN, in caps. Rehab is a cliche business—no pain, no gain.

Contract-relax stretching is very effective in relieving tension, regardless of its source. A form of strength training, it also helps to prevent muscle atrophy. Lay off the evil stuff like the *Clasp Knife* for awhile and stick to low intensity *Contrast Breathing* or *Forced Relaxation*. Do it many times throughout the day. Really focus on contracting and releasing the injured spot. You may apply pressure with your knuckles or fingertips as you flex the hurting unit.

Keep in mind that stretching is not a panacea, especially for the back. Those of you with bad backs, and if statistics do not lie, it is every other American, note on your forehead: stretching will relieve the pain, but will not fix you up.

Spasms and pain are only symptoms. The real problem is usually weakness. A weak back muscle has to contract hard just to keep you from walking on all fours—spinal erectors are 'anti-gravity muscles'. This tension is difficult to maintain, so the muscle just locks up. Movement and circulation become limited, so it gets even weaker, so it cramps even more to get even weaker to cramp even more... It's a vicious circle.

Conclusion: trying to fix a bad back with stretching is about as useful as an oil change on the *Titanic*. You'd better get on the first name basis with deadlifts. *Power to the People!: Russian Strength Secrets for Every American* will show you how.

The demographics of stretching

Your age and sex dictates your choice of stretching exercises, even more than your sports and activities. It is unfortunate that youth coaches and other people who should know better do not appreciate this simple fact.

Take girls' gymnastics, for instance. Russian scientist V. I. Fillipovich explains in his *Gymnastics Theory and Methodology* textbook:

"The obvious ease with which girl gymnasts master different exercises requiring maximal flexibility frequently encourage forcing the process of this quality's development. Its negative influence may not show immediately. Excessive emphasis on flexibility in young age may negatively affect the joints' strength, lead to a variety of spine deformities and have an unhealthy effect on postural development.

Flexibility development must be gradual. One must keep in mind that girl gymnasts frequently have a so-called active insufficiency. They cannot reach a great range of motion not for the lack of elasticity of the muscles and ligaments, but because of insufficient strength of the muscles that propel the movement. In other words, the existing anatomical mobility of the joints cannot be fully taken advantage of. It becomes quite obvious that one must work on simultaneous strength and flexibility development to reach a maximal movement amplitude."

Young girls should concentrate on the active stretches covered in my *Super Joints* book and video, sometimes to the exclusion of other methods.

Fillipovich goes as far as to state that children younger than ten or eleven, girls and boys, should not do any passive stretching at all; no contract-relax, no relaxed stretching, nothing of the sort!

It also makes sense from the psychological point of view: youngsters just do not have the patience and body control necessary for sophisticated methods such as *Forced Relaxation* or tedious ones such as *Waiting out the Tension*.

When it comes to kids, Fillipovich and other Soviet specialists especially warn against overstretching seven to ten year olds' shoulders—that includes pulling Junior by his arm when you are rushing him to the yellow bus—and spines, which are very vulnerable at this age.

In fact, until ten or eleven your gremlins should stay away from various forward and especially backward bends. Generally kids can be more aggressive with their hip and ankle joints though.

Youngsters should also be careful in their stretching and other athletic pursuits when undergoing the growth spurt. Adolescent hormones try their best to keep the ligaments pliable to accommodate the mushrooming bones, but the best is not always good enough.

Women who are pregnant, or who have had a child within a few months, should be especially careful with stretching. They should seek their doctor's advice. Delivery of a child requires extraordinary flexibility and the woman's body releases the hormone *relaxin* to loosen the ligaments. Relaxin is not selective, all the ligaments are affected. They will not tear easily, but will stretch beyond the norm leading to joint instability.

Most adults should focus on the contract-relax drills from this book to teach their stiff muscles to yield to stretches. Older folks also need isometric stretches, but they should emphasize the joint mobility drills from Super Joints. The idea is to lubricate and smooth out grindy joints.

Fast & Loose! is for everyone who wants to be flexible in motion and full of lazy relaxed energy, like a panther.

The details, the schedule

- Top Russian researcher Prof. Matveyev recommends that you perform isometric stretches—that covers *Contrast Breathing, Forced Relaxation*, and the *Clasp Knife*—in three to five sets per stretch four times a week. In my opinion it is a bit excessive. Most comrades will do fine on two to three days a week and two to three sets per stretch. The above is not writ in stone; experiment. It is good idea to make the sets in one workout progressively harder, at least some of the time.

- Do not get too much of a good thing. You are stretching too much, too hard, or too often if you get stiff and sore. Back off if you experience anything beyond very slight soreness the morning after.

- If you are ambitious about your splits, you could try Bill 'Superfoot' Wallace's hardcore stretching schedule: two intense stretching sessions a week and four easy ones. You could stretch isometrically on the two heavy days and wait out the tension on the light days.

- You do not need to do all the stretches on the list. Try them all if your health allows it, then pick and choose. Most comrades do not need much upper body stretching and should focus on their hamstrings and hip flexors first and foremost.

- The order of the stretches is not writ in stone, but you are advised to decompress your spine before stretching the hip flexors and stretch your groin after the hip flexors.

- If you perform the exercises from my other books, *Fast & Loose!* And *Super Joints*, rotate them in the following sequence:

Day 1	**Fast & Loose!**
Day 2	**Relax into Stretch**
Day 3	**Super Joints**

  Skip a day whenever you must and continue the rotation. The above recommendations are just the rules of thumb. Sophisticated trainers are encouraged to be creative.

• At least in the beginning you are advised to stay away from the *Clasp Knife technique*; *Contrast Breathing* and *Forced Relaxation* are safer choices.

• "Muscles should not be forced into any stretched position unless they have been previously warmed up through pre-loading," warned East German specialists J. Hartmann and H. Tunnemann. This may be a bit paranoid, but an isometric contraction held for up to a minute indeed brings in a pool of relaxing blood into the muscle. You do not need to do any special warm-ups; they are a total waste of time.

• Isometrics mess with your proprioceptors and impair your coordination for the rest of the day. So don't do them before your sport practice. The rule of thumb is: if you have to do a static stretch before you engage in your sport, you are not ready for the skill you are practicing. There are very few exceptions, for example, shoulder and wrist isometrics before squats for husky powerlifters who cannot get under the bar otherwise.

• Practice your *Relax into Stretch* exercises last, right after your workout or in the end of your day. Do not hit it too close too bed time if you can help it.

The *Relax into Stretch* drills—a quick reference

1. The Souped Up Toe Touch

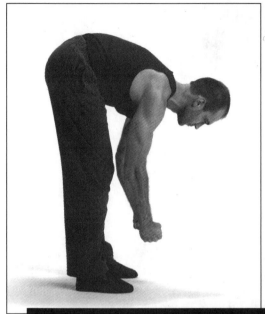

Slowly bend forward as far as it is comfortable for you.   No need to get ambitious yet.

Keep your knees locked or close to it and your weight balanced between your toes and your heels. Keep your head down and do not look up at all for the duration of the stretch.

Inhale—into your stomach if you know how—without popping up like a hydraulic jack. Squeeze your butt as hard as you can—imagine pinching a coin with your cheeks if you have trouble with that—and make white knuckle fists. Stay there for a second.

For some Comrades being upside down is hazardous. Ask your doctor if you are one of them.

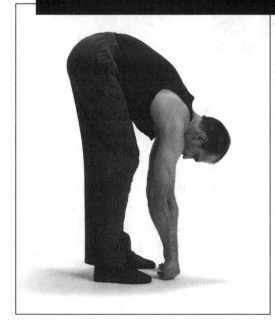

Release! —both the tension and the air at the same time. Remember the popped tire effect. If you listened like a good scout your body will drop down a little and stretch your backside: your hamstrings, your glutes, but mostly your lower back.

To fight hyperventilation and dizziness, wait a few moments before you inhale again.

Repeat the drill until you cannot go any deeper or some sort of discomfort—dizziness, a heavy head, strange sensations in your back, or whatever—hints at curtain time. For some folks being upside down is a plain bad idea; check with your doctor.

Once you have gone as deep as you can for the time being, bend your knees and go into a semi squat before standing up straight. It is essential for your back safety!

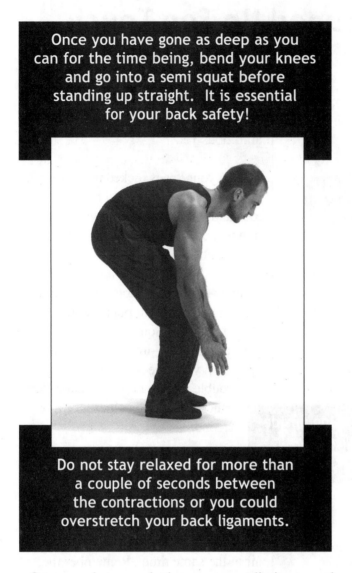

Do not stay relaxed for more than a couple of seconds between the contractions or you could overstretch your back ligaments.

Once you have reached your current limit or you have simply had enough, bend your knees and go into a semi squat before standing up straight. It is essential for your back safety!

Scientists found that when your spine is hyperflexed or very rounded, the lower back muscles just check out and leave all the work of supporting the spine to the ligaments. It means two things for you, Comrade. First, if you try to get up from the extremely bent over position using your back while keeping your legs straight, you are likely to get hurt. Second, because you are too smart to stretch your ligaments, you will not spend much time hanging relaxed between the contractions.

2. The Spine Decompression Hang

An acquaintance of mine, the chief detective of a police department in one of the former Soviet republics, was self-conscious about his height—or rather lack of it—and took up daily hanging from a pullup bar. His taller wife would wrap her arms and legs around his waist and hang on to him until his grip gave out.

The bizarre exercise paid off: the chap gained over an inch in height after a while.

Sandwiched between the vertebrae, your spinal discs act as shock absorbers. They hold water like sponges to do their job. Unfortunately, never-relenting gravity keeps squeezing the moisture out of them. The discs eventually dry out, get thin and brittle. Your spine shrinks, stiffens up, and becomes more injury prone.

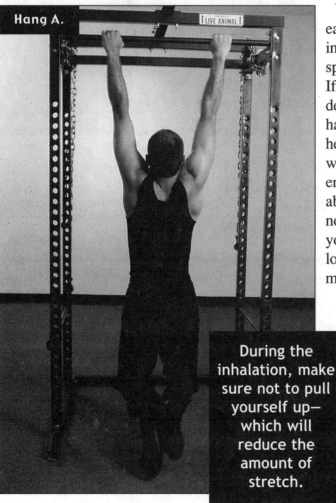

Hang A.

I LIVE ANIMAL I

During the inhalation, make sure not to pull yourself up—which will reduce the amount of stretch.

When astronauts return to earth they are a couple of inches taller than before the space flight, thanks to zero G. If NASA is not hiring, decompressing the spine by hanging from a pullup bar, head up, or upside down—as was the rage in the Bee Gees era—will allow the disks to absorb more moisture. It will not only help you reclaim your youthful height but will do a lot for your spinal health and mobility.

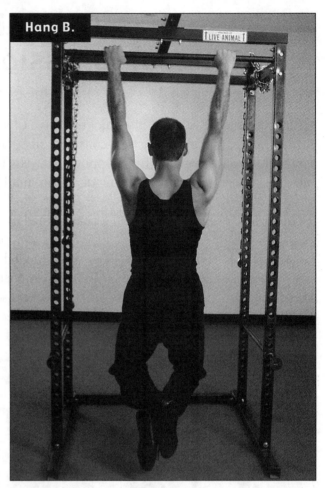

Hang B.

Plain old pullup bar hangs are alright, with or without the added weight of your spouse. Throw Contrast Breathing in the mix—and you will be blown away by the difference!

Hang from a pullup bar. If you are not strong enough to support your bodyweight, use one of those health club lat pulldown machines. If you cannot stand health clubs—you are not alone—hook sturdy bungy cords to the rafters in your basement, kneel on a folded towel, and hold on to the rubber bands.

Inhale deep and tighten every muscle in your body making sure that you do not pull yourself up (Hang A).

Hold your breath and the contraction for a moment, then suddenly let all the air go, along with the tension. You will drop and 'get taller' (Hang B).

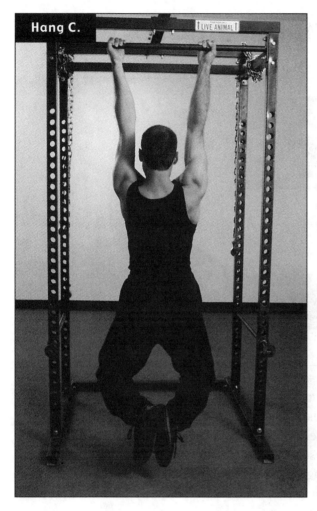

Hang C.

Repeat. Alternate your grips every time you perform the exercise—palms forward one time, palms back the next time. (Hang C).

Ideally, you should do this stretch every day throughout the day.

Still, twice a week is better than a slap on the face with a wet fish.

The spine extension and hip flexor stretches—and the splits—will groove a lot smoother, if you precede them with hanging back traction.

Make sure to hang out after lifting weights. A set of hangs after every set of deadlifts makes a healthy addition to the *Power to the People!* strength program.

3. The Improved Cobra

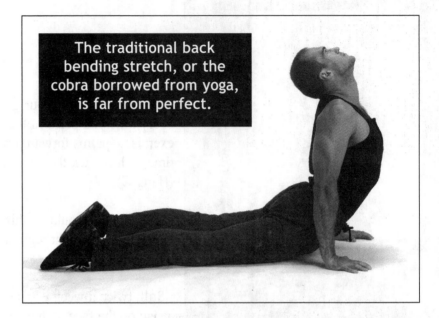

The traditional back bending stretch, or the cobra borrowed from yoga, is far from perfect.

The traditional back bending stretch, or the cobra borrowed from yoga, is far from perfect. First, many comrades, especially ladies, have a hard time supporting their weight in that position and therefore cannot concentrate on the stretch. Second, the length of your arms restricts the amount of stretch. Both problems are easily fixed if, instead of supporting your weight in the pushup position, you place your hands atop an object whose height matches your flexibility—be it a chair, the kitchen counter, or a training partner.

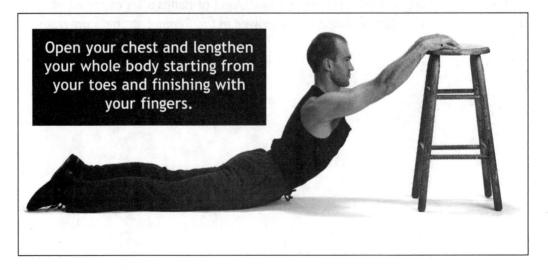

Open your chest and lengthen your whole body starting from your toes and finishing with your fingers.

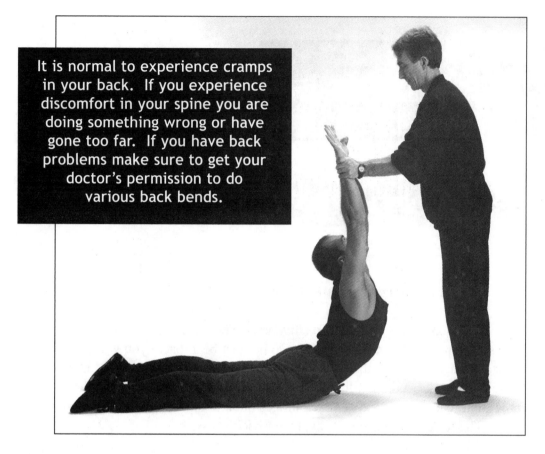

It is normal to experience cramps in your back. If you experience discomfort in your spine you are doing something wrong or have gone too far. If you have back problems make sure to get your doctor's permission to do various back bends.

Keep your arms and legs straight, point your toes, and open your chest. Elongate your spine, striving for the sensation you have experienced in the decompression hang. Go beyond stretching your spine; lengthen your whole body starting from your toes and finishing with your fingers. This maneuver opens up the spaces between the vertebrae and gives your discs and facet joints more room to play.

Inhale and flex your butt and abs. Flexing the abs means bracing them for a punch, not sucking them in or sticking them out. If you have a hard time getting it, a punch can be arranged.

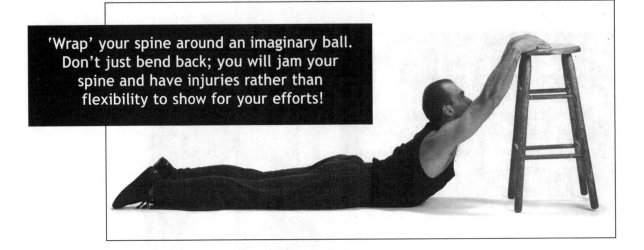

Release your breath and tension. Your hips will sag.

The improved cobra is a two-step stretch. The next step is to inhale and 'wrap' your spine around an imaginary ball.   Do not just bend back; you will jam your spine and have injuries rather than flexibility to show for your efforts! Unlike thoughtless back bending, 'elongating/wrapping around' does not limit the movement to a couple of lower back hinges but articulates the entire length of your spine. The result: greater flexibility, lower back stress.

Relax for a few seconds and repeat both steps: tension/release, followed by elongation/wrapping around.

It is normal to experience cramps in your back. If you experience discomfort in your spine or sacrum you are doing something wrong or have gone too far. Some comrades with back problems are not supposed to hyperextend their spines at all.

4. The Side Bend

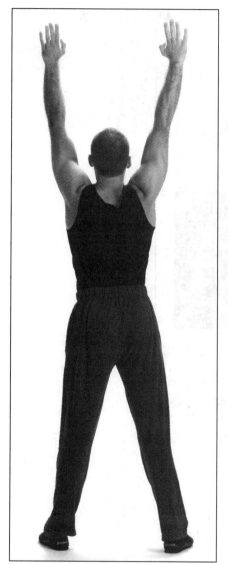

This goodie will stretch your side muscles and further decompress your spine, for that taller feeling.

Stand with your feet shoulder width and your knees locked. 'Grow tall' by reaching overhead (see photo to the left).

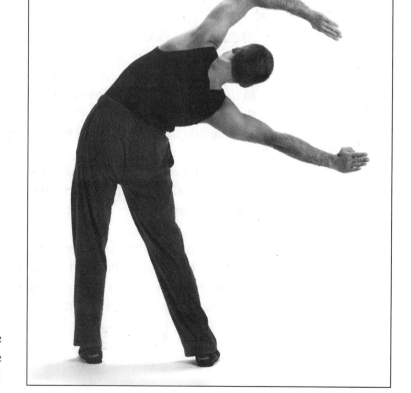

Lean strictly sideways as if you are sliding along a wall (see photo to the right). Do not twist!

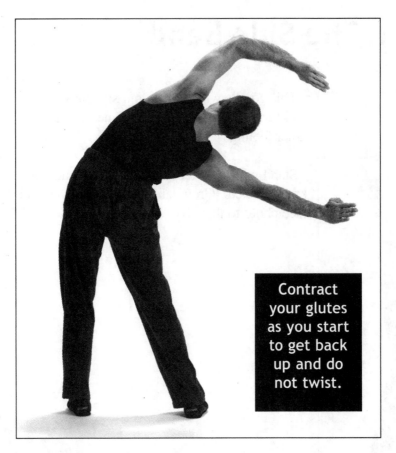

Contract your glutes as you start to get back up and do not twist.

Inhale and squeeze your butt tight. Whenever you have a hard time contracting a given muscle, flexing your glutes helps. Read up on the phenomenon of irradiation in *Power to the People!: Russian Strength Training Secrets for Every American* if you want to know why. Or just accept it as the ultimate truth; the Party is always right!

Let go in a second. Your body should fold slightly sideways without twisting. Your hips will move in the opposite direction to maintain the balance.

Once you cannot get any deeper in good form, squeeze your butt to get an irradiation boost, and slowly get up along the same path you have come down. If you do not flex your glutes you will be tempted to twist.

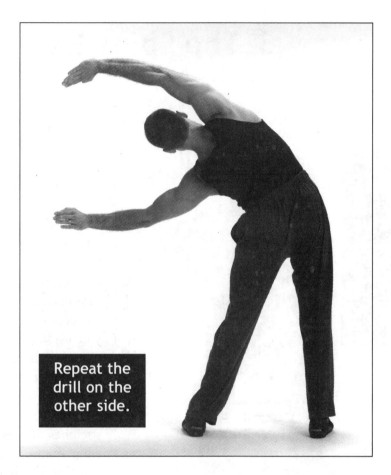

Repeat the drill on the other side.

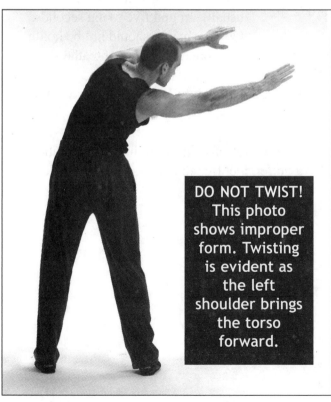

DO NOT TWIST! This photo shows improper form. Twisting is evident as the left shoulder brings the torso forward.

5. The Spine Rotation

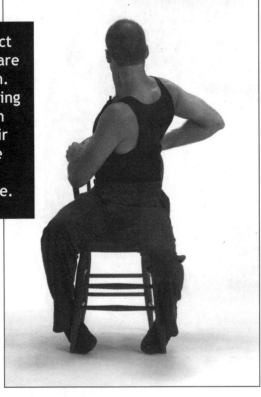

As usual, contract the muscles you are about to stretch. If you are stretching clockwise, push against the chair in the opposite direction: counterclockwise.

Sit upright in a chair with a stiff back. Solidly plant your feet to anchor your hips. Consider wrapping your feet around the legs of the chair.

Open your chest and turn your torso around your vertical spine. Hold on to the chair.

As usual, you shall contract the muscles you are about to stretch. If you are stretching clockwise as in the photo, push against the chair in the opposite direction: counterclockwise. Use your waist muscles; the arms just pass on the force. Unlike the previous stretches that respond to one-second contractions nicely, this drill usually calls for a longer time under tension—usually around five to ten seconds. Obviously you should not be holding your breath this long; breathe shallow.

Release the tension and air and increase the stretch by rotating further with the help of your arms. Do not slump over.

Keep at it, then switch sides. Your grand reward will be an increased rotational mobility in your spine. If you are a golfer, feel free to express your gratitude by putting me in your will.

6. The Lateral
Neck and Trap Stretch

Sit in a chair and grab it underneath the seat with your left hand.

Slowly lean your head and your body to the right. Keep your left arm straight. You should feel a stretch along the left side of your neck.

Place your right hand on the left side of your head as shown in the photo.

Push your hand and your head against each other for a while, anywhere from a few seconds to a minute if your neck is really tight. Breathe shallow.

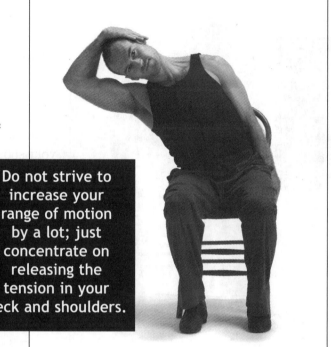

Do not strive to increase your range of motion by a lot; just concentrate on releasing the tension in your neck and shoulders.

Exhale and relax. Your neck will stretch further.

Repeat a few times. Do not strive to increase your range of motion by a lot; just concentrate on releasing the credit card tension in your neck and shoulders.

Repeat the drill on the other side.

If you have a muscle pull on, say, the left side of your neck, go easy on stretching the opposite, or right, side. When you stretch one muscle, its opposite number has to shorten. That's not a big deal unless the antagonist is injured; then it is likely to spasm. This rule applies all stretches. For example, if you have an injured hamstring and you ambitiously stretch your quad and hip flexor, the hammy will cramp and make you holler for your mommy.

7. The Headache Buster

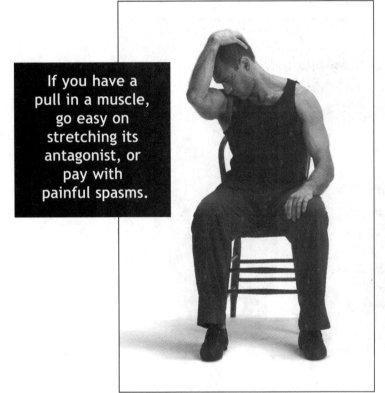

If you have a pull in a muscle, go easy on stretching its antagonist, or pay with painful spasms.

This variation of the previous stretch is the mother of all tension headache busters.

Turn your head a little to the right side as if trying to touch your collarbone with your chin. The left arm may be in any comfortable position. Better yet, place it behind your shoulder blades. Ideally, grab the right upright of the back of the chair if you can reach that far.

Apply the tension in the plane that crosses your left shoulder and right knee. Naturally, do the drill on both sides, always finishing with the tighter one.

8. The Anti-Slouch Neck Stretch

If you work with a computer or work at a desk, chances are the muscles in the front of your neck have shortened and given you a slouched posture.

This will also be the case if you do the dumbest ab exercise of all, the crunch. Say no to crunches and get on the *Bullet-Proof Abs* program! And do not forget to stretch your neck.

Before tackling the following stretch check with your doctor, especially if you have high blood pressure or neck problems. It is a great drill for some and bad news for others. This neck move has been my pet stretch since I got rear-ended by a semi and walked away alive, but without a neck curve. Thanks, Carl.

Lie on the edge of a bench or a sturdy table so your head hangs off the edge.

Inhale and tighten up your neck as if bracing for a punch.

Hold the tension and air for a second and release. Your head will drop a little. Repeat a few times as long as you do not experience discomfort. When you relax between the contractions try to decompress and elongate your cervical spine.

As an option, you may lift your head up a little, or till your chin touches your chest, on the inhalation. Then lower your head on a passive exhalation. Obviously, although you should be relaxed on the way down, exercise control so your head does not drop and whiplash!

9. The Head Turner

Here is the stretch for the comrades who have a hard time looking over their shoulders. Again, if you have an overly tight muscle on one side of your neck take it easy stretching the other side.

Sit in a chair as in the *Headache Buster* and turn your head as far as you can. Do not tilt your head! Just rotate it.

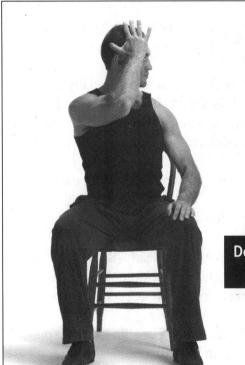

Apply pressure against your head with your hand. Hold the tension for some time without holding your breath.

Release and turn your head further. Use your neck muscles rather than your arm strength.

Perform the drill on both sides.

**Do not tilt your head!
Just rotate it.**

10. The Chest Opener

To stretch your pecs and open up your chest, stand inside a doorway and place your hands slightly below shoulder level. Instead of using a door you can have your training partner hold your wrists.

Your palms should be facing forward and your elbows must be slightly bent for the duration of the stretch. Carefully 'fall' forward and load your pectoral muscles. Be certain to lean with your whole body rather than just fold at the hips.

Inhale and build up the pressure against the doorway or your partner's hands. Exert the force as if you are trying to bring your palms together in front of you.

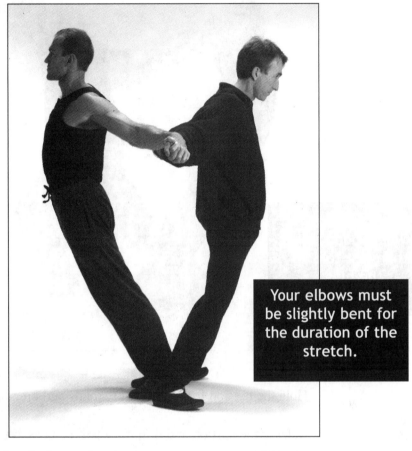

Your elbows must be slightly bent for the duration of the stretch.

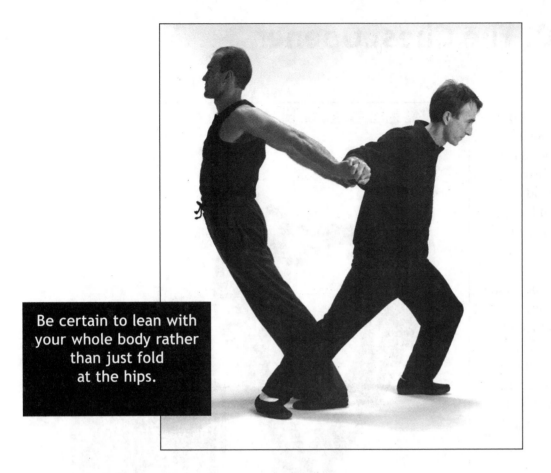

Be certain to lean with your whole body rather than just fold at the hips.

Hold the tension for five to ten seconds and breathe shallow.

Release the tension and drop forward on a passive exhalation. Drop your whole body rather than just your torso!

Repeat a few times. You rarely need to do more than one set of this stretch.

You can vary the stretching effect around your shoulder girdle by adjusting the height of your hand placement.

11. The Overhead Reach

Here is a crucial stretch for weightlifters and track & field athletes.

Get down on your knees and place your hands on an elevation, for example a chair, a kitchen counter, a power rack pin. Keep your elbows locked.

Press down against the chair. You should feel tension in your armpits and in the back of your arms.

Hold steady tension without holding your breath. Compared to other upper body stretches, this one may require a long time under tension, say 15-30 sec. Some comrades, especially those with well-developed shoulder girdle muscles, may need additional loading. Have your training partner apply steady pressure with his hand against the middle of your back.

Release and drop down. Gently increase the stretch even further by opening your chest and pushing it down.

Start with a very wide grip and narrow it to the shoulder width over a period of weeks and months.

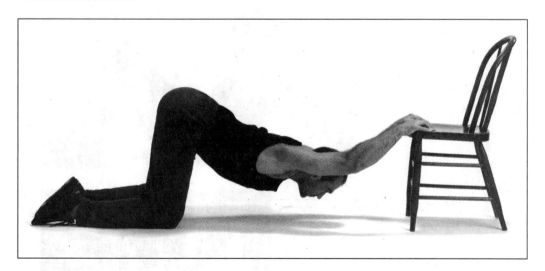

12. The Biceps and Shoulder Stretch

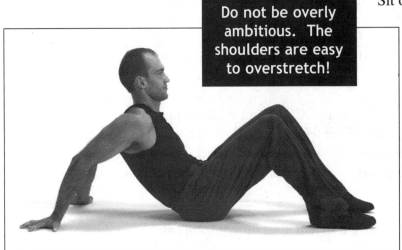

Do not be overly ambitious. The shoulders are easy to overstretch!

Sit on the floor with your knees bent and your arms behind you as shown. Keep your elbows slightly bent throughout the stretch.

With some weight on your palms apply pressure forward. It should feel like you are performing a biceps curl and are raising your arms in front of you at the same time. If you are a bodybuilder, imagine you are doing the Arnold curl.

Release. Your body will drop down and you will feel a stretch in your biceps and shoulders.

Carefully scoop your butt toward your feet and repeat the drill.

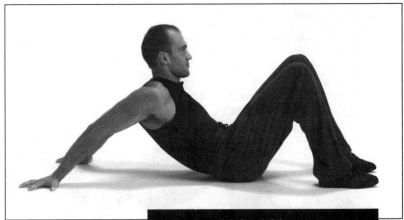

It should feel like you are performing a biceps curl and are raising your arms in front of you at the same time.

Do not be overly ambitious. The shoulders are easy to overstretch! If you feel pinpoint soreness in front of your shoulders the day after this stretch you have gone too far.

13. The Shoulder Blade and Lat Stretch

This awesome stretch will loosen up the tight muscles between your shoulderblades and stretch your lats—the muscles that fold like wings, downward from your armpits. Arnold Schwarzenegger used to do a variation of the following stretch to stimulate growth in his latissimus.

With your hands close together, hold on to a sturdy object at waist level. The doorknob on an open door is an option, if you are certain the door will not collapse under your weight. Face the edge of the open door and hold on to the knobs on both sides of it. Your feet should straddle the door under your hands.

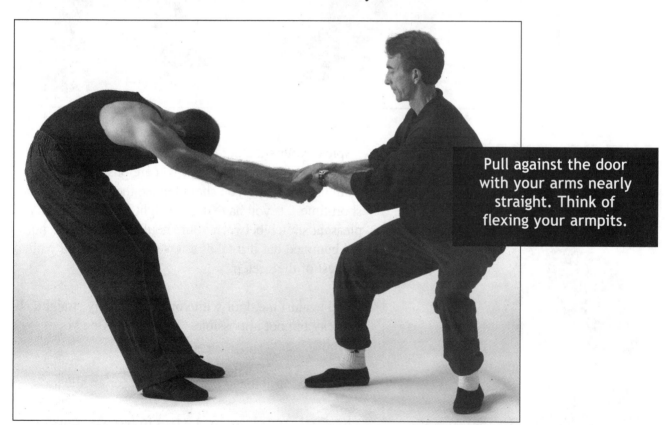

Pull against the door with your arms nearly straight. Think of flexing your armpits.

Stick your butt out and hang on the door while keeping your arms nearly straight, your head down, and your back rounded. Your knees should stay slightly bent throughout the drill.

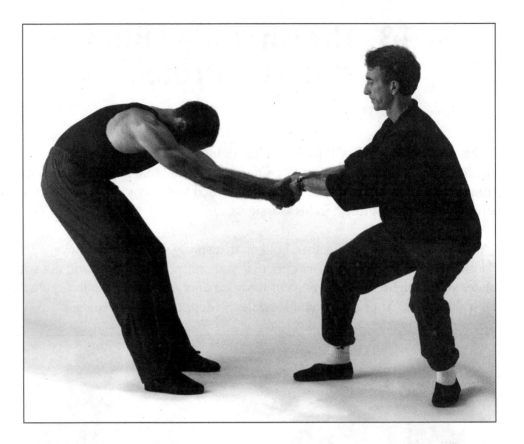

Spread your shoulder blades if you can. By humping your back and imagining that you are pushing away from the doorknob you should make them kick out in a short time. If you have done it right you should feel a pleasant stretch between your shoulder blades. Do not get bummed out if it takes a few weeks. Proceed with the rest of the stretch.

Pull against the door with your arms nearly straight! It is tricky but not impossible. Think of flexing your armpits.

Hold the tension and breath shallow for awhile.

Release! You should feel a pull from your armpits along and across your back. Kick out the shoulder blades again, or at least try to, before the next contraction.

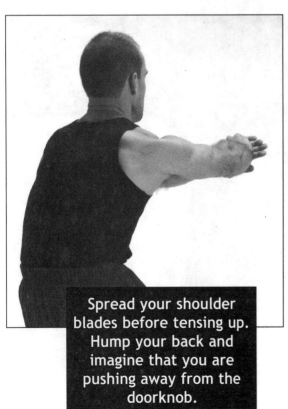

Spread your shoulder blades before tensing up. Hump your back and imagine that you are pushing away from the doorknob.

14. The Upper Back Loosener

This weird stretch will loosen up the muscles between your shoulder blades from a different angle and stretch out a tight upper back.

Hold on to the doorway or your training partner with one hand. Fold your free arm over the busy one. Keep your feet almost under your holding hand. If you do it right you will feel out of balance.

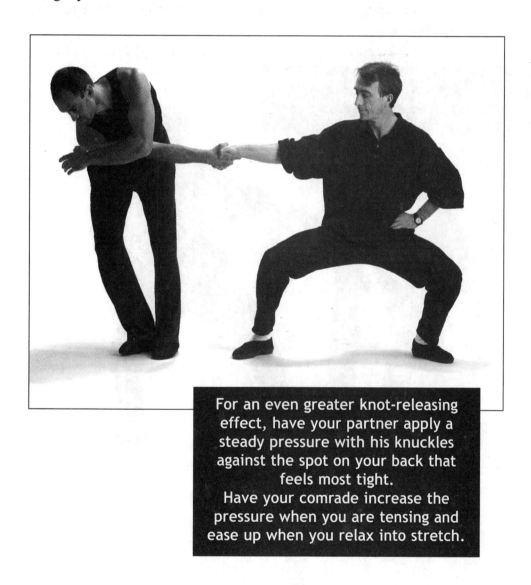

For an even greater knot-releasing effect, have your partner apply a steady pressure with his knuckles against the spot on your back that feels most tight.
Have your comrade increase the pressure when you are tensing and ease up when you relax into stretch.

Lean away over and away from the holding hand. Experiment with the direction of the bend and the height of the holding hand. You will notice that by changing the loading angle you can stretch any spot on your upper back with great precision.

Pull with a straight arm against the doorknob or your assistant's hand.

Release and feel the stretch where you have never felt it before!

For an even greater knot-releasing effect have your partner apply a steady pressure with his knuckles against the spot on your back that feels most tight. Have your comrade increase the pressure when you are tensing and ease up when you relax into stretch.

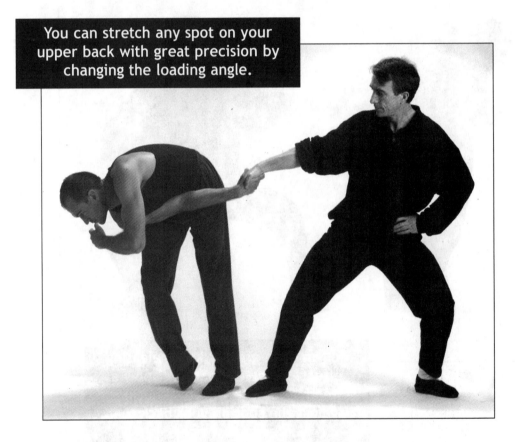

You can stretch any spot on your upper back with great precision by changing the loading angle.

15. The Wrist Flexion

Get down on your knees and place your hands in front of you, fingers pointing towards you as much as possible. Keep your elbows locked for the duration of the stretch.

Gently shift some weight on your hands until you feel a pull on the inside of your forearms.

Apply pressure against the ground as if trying to straighten out your wrists. Since your forearm muscles sport good endurance, hold the tension for a relatively long time, at least ten seconds.

The angle between your hands and your arms will increase when you have released the tension.

Be careful not to overdo this stretch! It is way too easy to damage the wrists. My arm-wrestling buddies, stay the hell away from this stretch!

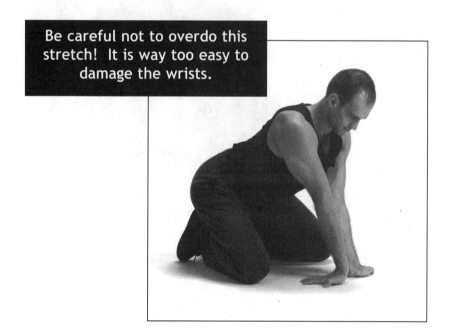

Be careful not to overdo this stretch! It is way too easy to damage the wrists.

16. The Wrist Extension

Assume the same position as in the last stretch, except rest on the backsides of your palms. Keep your elbows locked for the duration of the stretch.

Experiment with the direction where your fingers point; turn them slightly in and then out and note the effect on your forearms.

Contract the muscles on the outside of your forearms, as if trying to stand up on your finger tips.

Release, and increase the stretch by gently shifting your body back.

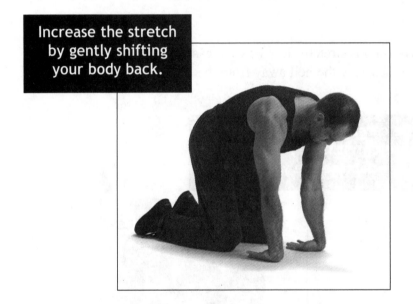

Increase the stretch by gently shifting your body back.

17. The Good Morning Hamstring Stretch

Bending forward with a barbell on your shoulders is one of the key exercises in weightlifting and powerlifting. For some mysterious reason, it is called 'a good morning'. As my friend and powerlifting champion, Marty Gallagher, has wondered: "Why does such a manly drill have such a 'hearts and flowers' name?"

This stretch closely mimics the Barbell Good Morning which makes it the first choice for an iron rat's hamstrings.

Even if you do not lift anything heavier than your laptop, make this your first hammy stretch because it will finally teach you the difference between stretching your back and stretching your hamstrings. Few comrades get the difference, hence many overstretched backs and overly tight hams.

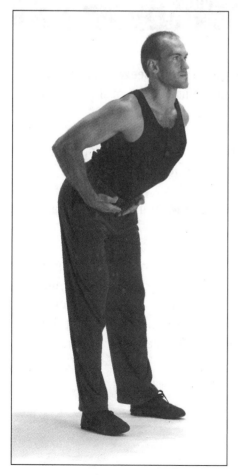

Stand normally, your feet shoulder width apart and pointing forward. Start by placing the edges of your hands into the creases on top of your thighs. I learned this neat trick from a friend of my wife's, dance instructor Kathy Foss Bakkum. Press your hands hard into your 'hinges' and stick your butt out while keeping your weight on your heels. Your knees should be slightly bent.

Keep your chest open, your lower back arched, and your chin pointed forward throughout this and other hamstring stretches! If you do not, your hammies will remain forever tight.

As you are folding, you will feel a pull right underneath your butt—or a hand's width above your knees. If you do not—read the manual again! Once you have understood what a hamstring stretch is supposed to feel like, reach your arms forward for balance and finally get to work!

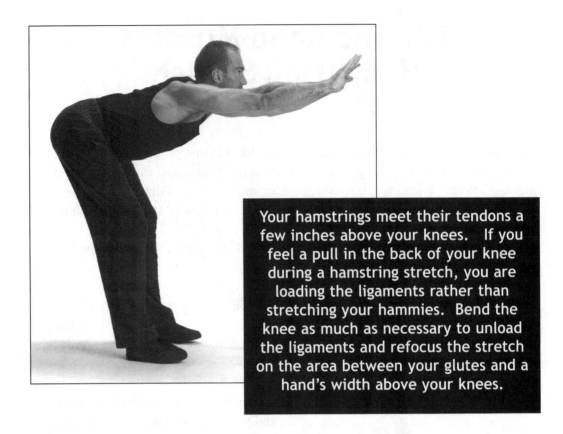

Your hamstrings meet their tendons a few inches above your knees. If you feel a pull in the back of your knee during a hamstring stretch, you are loading the ligaments rather than stretching your hammies. Bend the knee as much as necessary to unload the ligaments and refocus the stretch on the area between your glutes and a hand's width above your knees.

Flex the spots where you feel the pull. At the same time squeeze your butt and imagine that you are trying to paw the ground with your heels or push your heels through the floor.

When you release the tension your body will fold like a jackknife. Appreciate the difference between folding like a jackknife and bending forward!

Naturally, you cannot completely relax with the Good Morning stretch because your back must stay straight and your chin up.

After this relative relaxation increase the stretch even more by sticking your butt even further back and, if you know how, contracting your hip flexors—the muscles in the front hinges you have pushed against with your hands. It does not hurt to have a spotter in case you overbalance and keel over. Holding on to something for balance and/or having a wall behind you to break the fall, is another option

If you are still afraid to do the drill standing, you may practice it sitting on the edge of a very sturdy chair. Sitting on the floor will not give you the necessary leverage unless you are already super flexible.

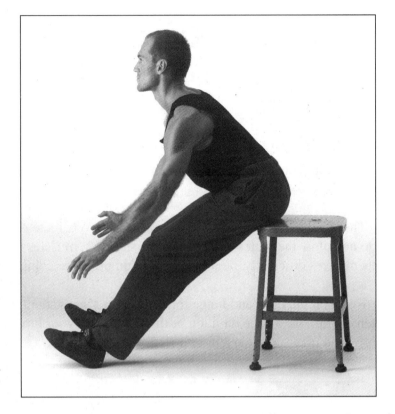

To avoid creating a flexibility imbalance in various muscles on the back of your legs, do not let your feet roll out but point your toes straight ahead or up. There's nothing to it with the Standing Good Morning, because your feet are anchored. But if you choose the Seated Good Morning, you will have to pay attention.

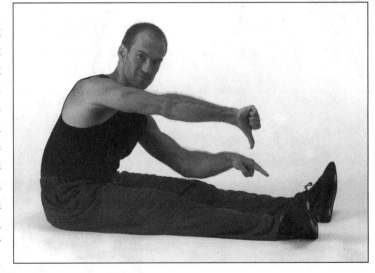

18. The Kneeling Hip Flexor Stretch

Tight hip flexors are the culprit behind bad backs, monkey butts, and athletic mediocrity.

The hip flexors are your glutes' antagonists. When the hip flexors are tight, they do not allow the glutes—which are the strongest muscles in your body—to exert themselves efficiently, be it in running, jumping, punching, or any other activity.

Kneel on the floor and lunge forward. Your torso and the front shin should remain upright for the duration of the stretch and your hips should stay squared off. You may spot yourself with chairs if you wish.

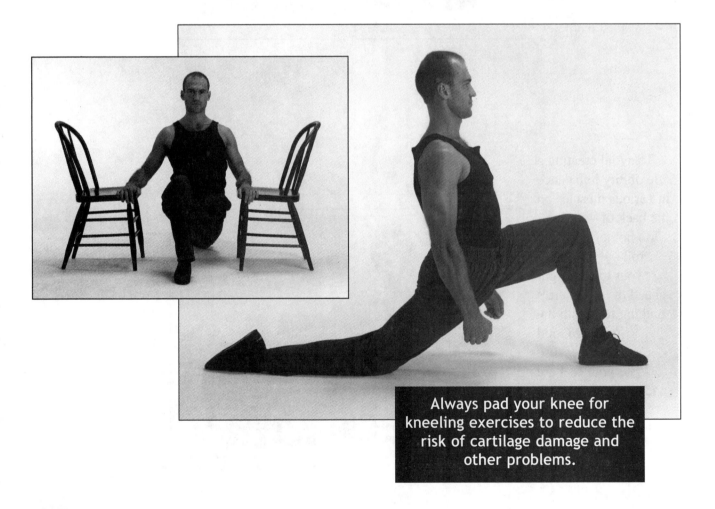

Always pad your knee for kneeling exercises to reduce the risk of cartilage damage and other problems.

Flex your abs to protect your back and contract the hip flexors—the muscles on the front of the kneeling leg—by imagining that you are going to kick forward with that foot or knee.

Once you release the tension, you will sag straight down. It is imperative for success and safety. Leaning forward, placing your hands on your knee, letting your knee drift forward, and twisting are out! Make a point of looking out and not down because your body tends to follow your head.

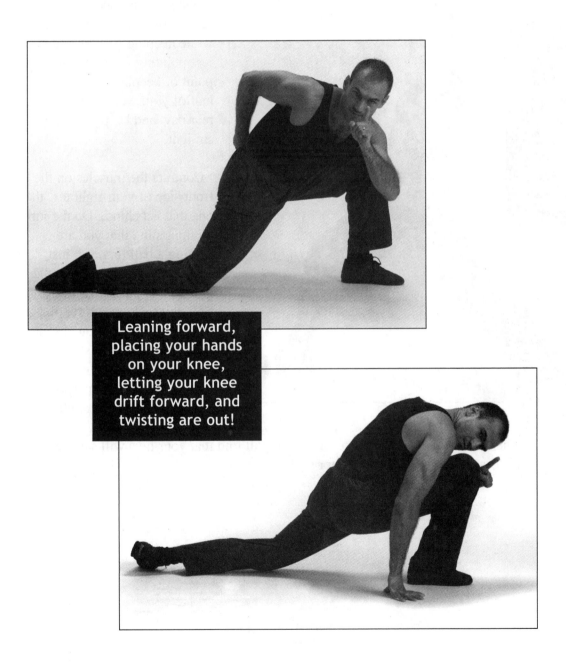

Leaning forward, placing your hands on your knee, letting your knee drift forward, and twisting are out!

19. The Lunge Hip Flexor Stretch

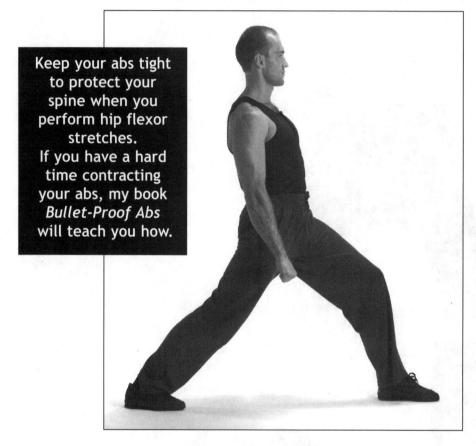

Keep your abs tight to protect your spine when you perform hip flexor stretches.
If you have a hard time contracting your abs, my book *Bullet-Proof Abs* will teach you how.

This stretch is an alternative to the kneeling one. Take a reasonably wide step forward while keeping both of your feet pointing forward. Make a point of keeping more than half of your weight on your rear paw and keep the latter straight.

Contract the muscles on the front side of your right leg, the one that is behind. Do the job by imagining that you are kicking a ball forward; just 'suck' your back foot into the ground and push forward. You will feel tension running down your quad. You abs are tight. Make sure to stay totally upright; leaning forward defeats the purpose of all the karate stance stretches.

When you have let go of the tension, you will find that your hips will sag and shift forward slightly. Still stay upright!

Now imagine that you are a fencer performing a lethal lunge and slowly propel yourself forward by pushing off your straight rear leg (Right).
Do not twist; make sure that your body is facing straight ahead. I shall be redundant: do not lean forward.

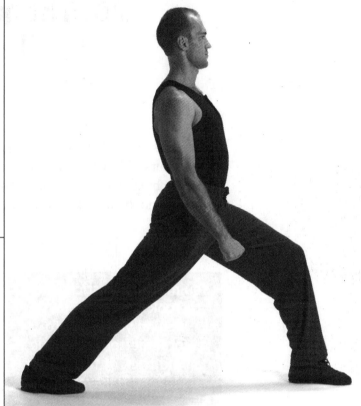

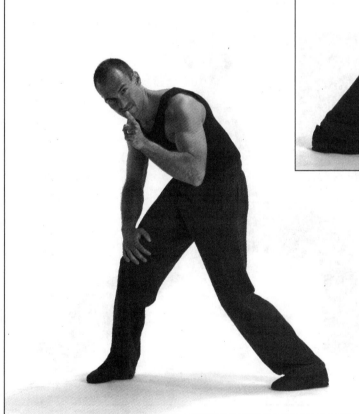

Keep repeating as far as you maintain good form: an upright back and the front shin, squared off hips and torso, both feet pointing forward, the knees track their feet and do not bow in. If you look something like this (Above)—you will have many injuries and zero flexibility! It is OK if your heel slightly comes off the floor though.

20. The Karate Stance
Hip Flexor Stretch

Stretch as you did previously: apply forward pressure with the rear leg, then propel yourself forward with the same leg. Now, you will feel the stretch not only at the hip hinge but also in the groin. To be safe, make certain that your back knee is locked and the muscles surrounding it are contracted.

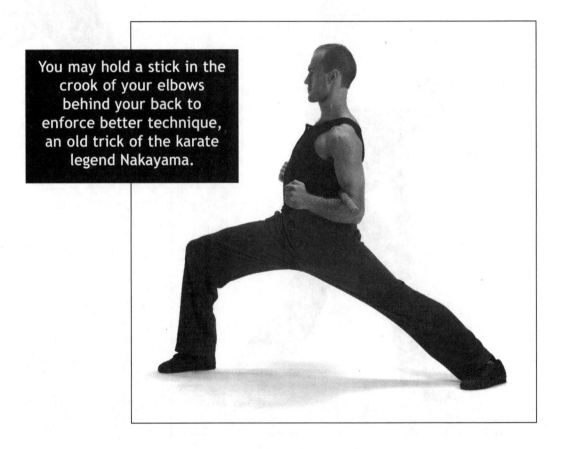

You may hold a stick in the crook of your elbows behind your back to enforce better technique, an old trick of the karate legend Nakayama.

Your rear foot should maintain a surface contact with hundred percent of its surface. Unfortunately, at an extreme angle, this drill becomes hard on the ankle. That is why you should advance to a different stretch, for example, the intermediate groin stretch, before you reach that level. A possible exception is a karateka who makes an informed choice to keep on advancing in this highly karate-specific stretch, in spite of possible health risks.

Do not think that these drills benefit only karatekas, however. I teach this and the following stretch to powerlifters who have a hard time locking out their deadlifts and I cannot think of a sport where they would not be helpful.

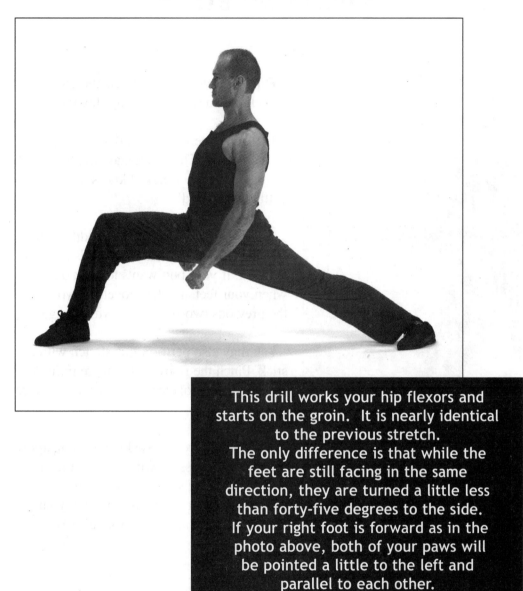

This drill works your hip flexors and starts on the groin. It is nearly identical to the previous stretch.
The only difference is that while the feet are still facing in the same direction, they are turned a little less than forty-five degrees to the side.
If your right foot is forward as in the photo above, both of your paws will be pointed a little to the left and parallel to each other.

21. The Karate Stance Groin Stretch

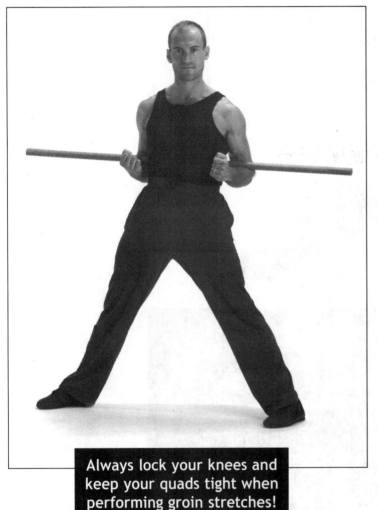

Always lock your knees and keep your quads tight when performing groin stretches!

This drill, although it targets the groin muscles, also works your hip flexors.

This time keep your feet flat and parallel to each other. The knees stay tightly locked for the duration. Relaxed knees are prone to getting wrenched!

Do not be aggressive on the width of the stance. Make sure that your pelvis is thrust forward. If your butt wants to stick out even when your feet are close together, work on the previous two stretches a while longer.

You may also perform this stretch with a stick. Pinch the floor as if you are trying to slide your feet together or are trying to close scissors.

When you have released the tension, apply the outward pressure with your feet (as if you are opening scissors). At no point should your feet roll in or out; keep your 'suction cups' flat on the ground!

As you apply the outward pressure, slowly turn your hips in one direction, and then another. At no point should your butt stick out! You should have a solid, grounded, powerful feeling and your torso will remain upright.

After a few repetitions carefully take a wider step and repeat the drill. I repeat, do not go too wide—to avoid overstretching the outside of your ankles!

Once you have progressed to what you believe is your safe limit, it is a good idea to periodically practice all the karate stance stretches in the maintenance mode—for the powerful body awareness effect they offer for any sport. Perhaps you could do one set of these stretches before your splits.

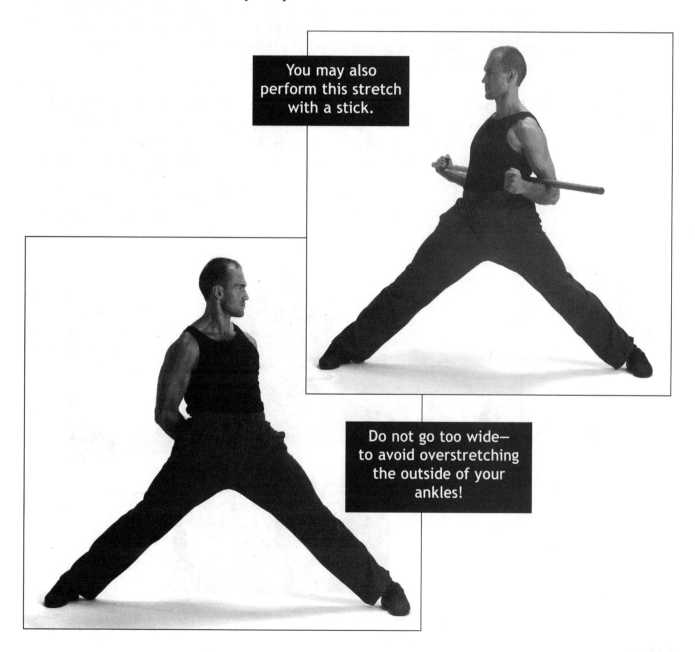

You may also perform this stretch with a stick.

Do not go too wide—to avoid overstretching the outside of your ankles!

22. The Seated Groin Stretch

Sit on the floor and place something moderately slippery under your feet. If you exercise on a carpet, glossy magazine covers work well. Thick socks are good on a vinyl mat, and you cannot do better than folded wash clothes for hardwood. Skateboards are to be avoided.

Spread your legs as wide as you comfortably can (don't worry, comfort will end very soon). If you cannot sit with your legs straight and spread and your back insists on staying rounded you are not ready for this drill! Work on your good mornings and karate stretches for awhile before tackling this one.

Place your hands behind your back and gently lift yourself up. Open your chest as much as possible and imagine that you are trying to push the walls apart with your feet. This imagery—recommended by Moscow hand-to-hand combat instructor Vlad Fadeyev—will enable you to immediately increase your stretch by a couple of inches!

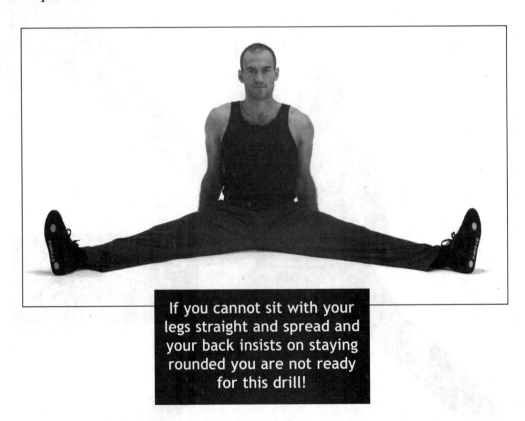

If you cannot sit with your legs straight and spread and your back insists on staying rounded you are not ready for this drill!

When the walls refuse to move any further, gingerly lower your butt to the floor. Keeping your chest up, carefully push your belly forward until you feel tension in your inner thighs. Do not round your back. Keep your hands in front of you, but do not touch the ground unless you are heading for trouble and need a spot. Make sure that your toes are pointing to the ceiling and do not flop outward, now or at any point during this stretch!

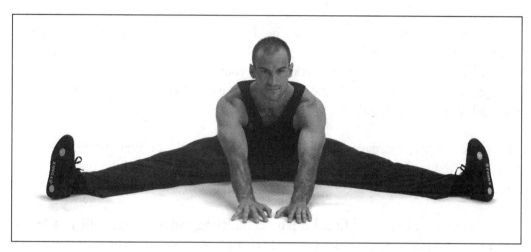

Contract your tight inner thighs. If you have a hard time getting your adductors to tense up, you have either found some sneaky way of keeping the weight off them (knock it off, before I order you to do pushups!), or you are not ready for this stretch yet. If you cannot spread your legs far enough apart to start with, you will not generate enough leverage. Swallow your pride and go back to the karate stretches.

Hold the tension for a period of time determined by the variation of the contract-relax stretching you are employing. I personally prefer Forced Relaxation and a roughly twenty-second contraction for this stretch.

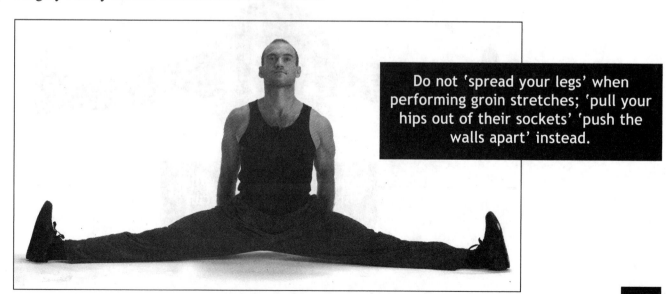

Do not 'spread your legs' when performing groin stretches; 'pull your hips out of their sockets' 'push the walls apart' instead.

When you finally release the tension with a sigh of relief your limp body will drop forward a little. Your hands may now touch the floor and catch your weight. It is good to use your hands to limit your advance to small increments for increased safety. Be certain to keep your lower back reasonably straight throughout the stretch to increase the effectiveness of the drill and to avoid overstretching the back ligaments!

Flex your adductors again and repeat the drill. You may experience slight pain inside your knees. If you have done everything like I told you and you doctor has assured you that there is nothing wrong with your knees, here is what you should do. Concentrate the tension on the tender spots and hold it for long periods of time, 30-60 seconds, before releasing.

Do not attempt to increase the ROM for a while—weeks or even months. Keep on practicing long contractions without stretching advances, until the tissues around your knees get stronger and stop bothering you.

If, or once, your knees are fine, keep on contracting and relaxing, until your trunk either does not move any further forward without excessive rounding, or the whole thing gets really old. Now it is time to carefully sit up, shift your weight on your hands behind you, and push the walls apart again. Then lean forward and repeat the whole sequence. Once your ROM stops increasing or you start contemplating my murder, slowly get out of the stretch.

You may want to do a set or two in Waiting out the Tension style, before starting your isometric stretching sets.

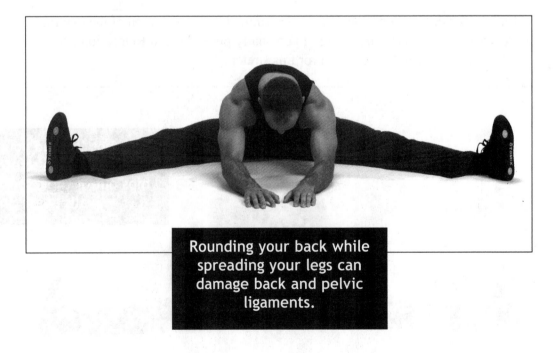

Rounding your back while spreading your legs can damage back and pelvic ligaments.

23. The Calf Stretch

Assume the pushup position on the floor—or against a sturdy elevation if you find the floor stretch too difficult for the time being. Shift your weight to the balls of your feet. Your knees may be slightly bent.

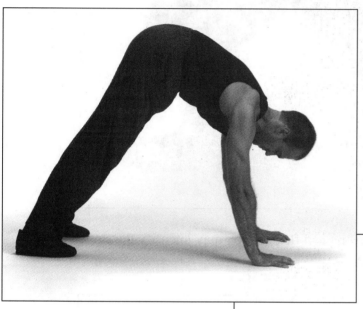

Tighten up your calves by imagining that you are trying to get up on your tiptoes. Hold steady tension for a long time—calves boast spectacular endurance—before releasing it.

Use a sturdy elevation if you find the floor stretch too difficult for the time being.

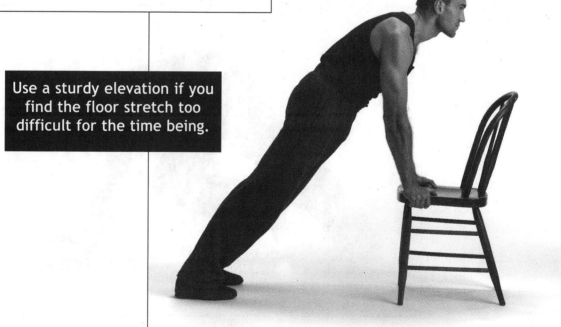

Let your body slip forward from the knees up, while keeping your heels in contact with the floor. The angle between your shins and your feet will get smaller. Repeat for the appropriate number of contractions.

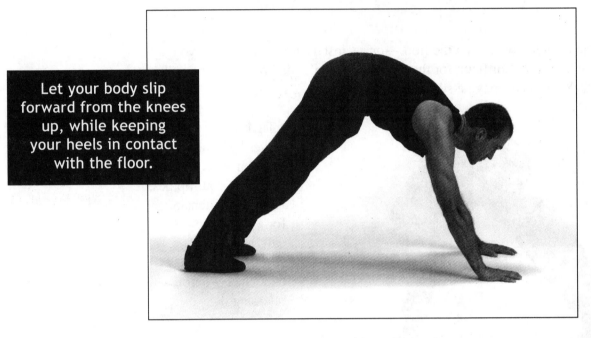

Let your body slip forward from the knees up, while keeping your heels in contact with the floor.

Once your calves are strong and flexible you may intensify the stretch by working one leg at a time.

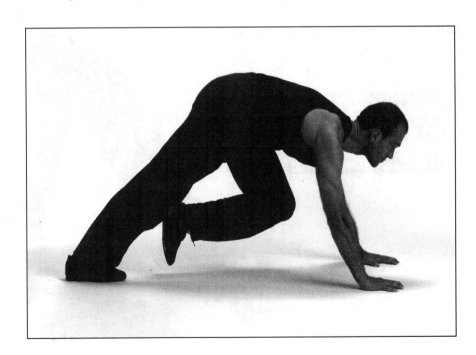

24. The Shin and Instep Stretch

Are the muscles on your shins tight from running? Do you want to be able to point your toes better for kickboxing or dancing? Then this foot-flexion stretch is for you.

Sit on your heels with your toes pointed back.   If your knees refuse to hyperflex painlessly, stick a stiff pillow or something similar between your hamstrings and your calves, to limit knee bending.

Shift your weight back. If you lean forward you will fail to stretch the target area. Contract the muscles on your shins by pushing with your insteps against the floor, as if you are trying to bring your toes towards your knees.

When you release the tension, your body will sink a little, as your feet move toward being in a straight line with your shins.

Now point your toes even more—as if someone is pulling you by your toes and is trying to pull your ankles out of their sockets.

Repeat the whole sequence as many times as necessary.

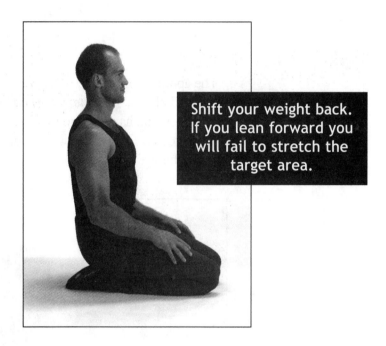

Shift your weight back. If you lean forward you will fail to stretch the target area.

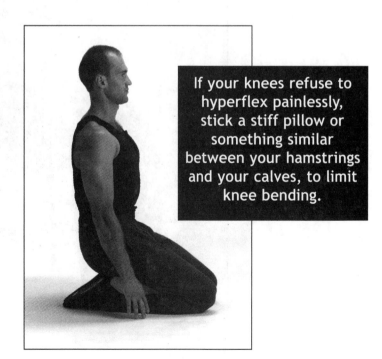

If your knees refuse to hyperflex painlessly, stick a stiff pillow or something similar between your hamstrings and your calves, to limit knee bending.

Most of the above stretches are demonstrated on the companion video, *Relax into Stretch.*

The application of *Relax into Stretch* technique is not limited to the stretches described above. You can creatively solve most unusual flexibility needs with the techniques you have learned. For instance, a martial artist who needs to be able to pull his toes back to protect them during barefoot front kicks can press his toes against the wall.

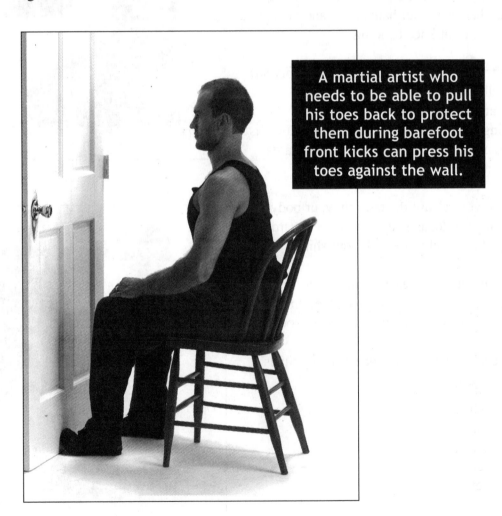

A martial artist who needs to be able to pull his toes back to protect them during barefoot front kicks can press his toes against the wall.

How much flexibility do you really need?

We did it for Britain and for the hell of it.

*—Richard Noble, on breaking
the world automobile absolute speed record*

Is flexibility always good? Can you be too flexible?

Americans don't think so. They stretch just for the sake of stretching. They just can't get enough.

Sorry to burst your bubble. Soviet research demonstrated that you need only a small flexibility reserve above the demands of your sport or activity. Excessive flexibility can be detrimental to athletic performance.

A classic Soviet text, *The Theory and Methodology of Physical Education,* warns: "One must remember that in some cases excessive flexibility not only does not help the athlete's technique, but interferes with it by 'dispersing' the acting forces (for example, a very flexible spine and a relaxed torso when taking off for a jump)."

Old school strongmen instinctively avoided stretching. They felt they could lift more weight if they stayed 'tight'. They were right. The stretch reflex fired sooner, making them more prone to an injury, but helping them to move more iron.

Russian Olympic weightlifters avoid full range movements of the muscles surrounding the hip and knee joints. Too much flexibility in that area makes the lifter sink too deep when he is getting under the barbell. The same is true for powerlifting. Fortunately, powerlifters, as a group, are least influenced by the pop fitness culture's deification of relaxed stretching, high carb/low fat/low protein diet, and other stupid ideas.

That is not to say that powerlifters do not need flexibility. They do—but no more than necessary to lift in good form. For example, tight hamstrings 'tuck your butt under'. As a result, back strength is wasted on fighting against your own hams, rather than the weight, in the squat and deadlift.

Soviet researcher, weightlifting champion, and coach Robert Roman determined that an athlete loses 15% of his pulling strength when he lifts with a rounded, rather than a flat back. That could mean the difference between first and last place!

Also, your hamstrings or back are likely to get injured. Hamstrings take forever to heal, but it is not the end of the world. The back is a more serious matter. A properly arched spine can support ten times more weight than a straight one, and even more than a rounded one. Ever heard a disk blow out? Sounds like a high tension cable going boink!

The lesson is not to stretch your hams until you can tie your shoes with your teeth, but just enough to maintain a tight arch in the 'hole', the bottom of the squat.

Whatever your sport, pay careful attention to the effect more flexibility has on your performance. Up to a point, your game will improve through increased efficiency of movement and less frequent injuries. Beyond that point you are in the red.

In sprinting, good spine rotation is needed for optimal technique—but an excessively loose trunk does not allow you to take full advantage of the pumping action of the arms.

In shot put or boxing, a super flexible waist will absorb the leg and hip drive instead of transferring it to the shoulder.

Even in a sport like kickboxing, one can get too flexible. When we finished our presentations at the Arnold Schwarzengger's Martial Arts Seminar, Bill 'Superfoot' Wallace told me over a hamburger that at one point he had worked up to a two hundred ten degrees negative side split (a classic split is one hundred and eighty degrees). The champion kickboxer's hips got so loose that he started having trouble snapping his kicks back after they had made contact with the target. That is when Superfoot pulled the plug on excess and decided that normal, straight line, splits are enough.

Never use flexibility to compensate for poor technique. Bodybuilders often complain how limited ankle flexibility affects their squat. Sorry, boys, when you squat properly, the movement in the ankle is minimal and you should be able to squat wearing ski boots. Learn to squat from a lifter and do not waste your time in a ballet class.

If you do not play sports and stretch just for health and the hell of it, it is up to you to decide how far you want to go. Just make sure that you have a small reserve of flexibility beyond the requirements of your lifestyle and check with a medical professional that you have no postural problems due to muscle tightness.

Expect that you will be more flexible in some areas than others. The ability to do a split does not automatically qualify you to do a competition style snatch. Having flexible hips does not imply mobile shoulders. The combo of an overstretched back and tight hamstrings is more widespread than high cholesterol.

Flexibility developed with one exercise does not always improve the range of motion of the same joint when tested in other exercises. In one study a group of subjects trained the toe-reach standing, and the other seated. Those who stretched in the seated position did not do well when they were tested standing. The other group did well on both tests. Go figure.

Conclusion: the transfer of training effect is inconsistent. Sometimes you have it, sometimes you don't. The fact that, say, the sit-and-reach is a part of the standard flexibility test is meaningless. I taught an NFL player how to cheat on that test and have no guilty conscience whatsoever.

If a stretch does not improve your game or make you feel better—lose it.

To sum up: develop some flexibility reserve beyond the demands of your sport and lifestyle, then keep on going as long as more mobility does not start having an adverse effect on your game.

I will either teach you how to do splits—or I will talk you out of it. No more guilt, Comrade!

When flexibility is hard to come by, build strength

If excessive flexibility is not your problem, rather the other way around, here is a couple of plateau-busting strategies.

First, get stronger. Typically a stronger muscle does not have to contract as hard as a weaker one to exert the same amount of force—and it more willingly relaxes into a stretch. If you hit a plateau with Forced Relaxation or other iso stretches, you should stop trying to increase the range for a while and concentrate instead on building strength.

Push harder. More importantly, push longer. When McDonagh and Davies reviewed the results of many studies of isometric strength training, they found out that variables such as the intensity of the contraction and the training frequency did not seem to matter much. The single common item in all successful programs was the high total time under tension in all the sets (e.g. TUT = 3 sets x 3 contractions x 30 seconds long = 270 sec).

Obviously, you can bump up the TUT by doing more contractions, more sets, or simply increase the tension holding time in your Forced Relaxation or *Clasp Knife* stretches.

Even if you are not at a standstill, where the going gets tough near the end of the stretch, it is a good idea not to up the ROM after every contraction. Try every other repetition. And make a habit of holding tension in the final stretched position for thirty seconds, as recommended by Prof. Leonid Matveyev.

Two more plateau busting strategies from the iron world

If they did [call me a sissy because I studied ballet], I'd stomp 'em and do a pirouette on their heads.

—Ken Avery, Cincinnati Bengals linebacker

Once you have mastered muscle length and tension control, it is hard to lose it. Although it is not quite as permanent as riding a bike—according to Popenko's data, your flexibility decreases by 10-20% in two months of no stretching—it is possible to maintain a high degree of flexibility in just two to three sessions a month.

Mike Song, a rock climber from Minneapolis who did his first split a couple of weeks after he took my seminar was too busy to train for a month afterwards. To his surprise, he went all the way into a full split the first time he tried it after the layoff! In fact, occasional time off will help you to improve due to the *reminiscence effect*.

In 1984 Jerry Moffat, the world's top rock climber from England, called it quits and rode into the sunset on his motorcycle. Nobody expected miracles from Jerry when he returned to the rock two years later. Yet two weeks after his comeback the supposed has-been climbed the best performance of his career!

Motor-learning experts know that a skill tends to improve after a layoff, the so-called *reminiscence effect*. Multiple repetitions of a drill, a rock climbing technique, a reverse punch, a split, or a deadlift, forms what Russians call the *dynamic stereotype*, or a 'how-to manual' of this movement in the athlete's nervous system. You learn to perform exactly as practiced—the form, the force, the range of motion, etc.

Although forming a dynamic stereotype is necessary to master a sports skill, once it is formed, it is difficult to improve on. Once you have reached a plateau, continued practice only reinforces it, which is why a powerlifter has to start all over with lighter weights once he has set a new personal best.

If you lay off stretching, your brain gets a chance to forget your limit. This is the essence of the reminiscence effect. Once your old PR has been erased, you are ready to train for a new one!

Russian author, Victor Popenko, advocates another plateau-busting strategy similar to a layoff—the *stepwise progression*.

It is known that, in any endeavor, it takes much less effort to maintain the achieved performance level than to reach it in the first place. Say, you have been practicing splits for five sets three times a week. You have made good progress but finally hit the wall. Then cut back to the minimal amount of stretching which maintains your current level, for example two sets once every five days.

Maintenance requirements vary from person to person. I can skip up to a month and still do a split in a seminar through shear grit. Most comrades need to practice at least once every five to seven days, lest they choose to slide back. Having stabilized your flexibility for a few weeks, once again increase your training load—and exceed your old limits!

It is interesting that, while the layoff strategy is similar to powerlift cycling, Popenko's stabilization backoff is similar to the Bulgarian and Chinese weightlifters' practice of reducing the volume of their lifting by 40% every fourth week.

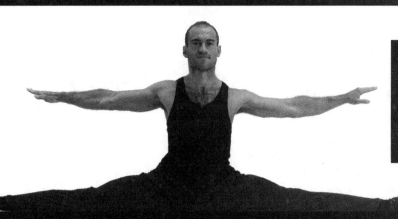

Once you get proficient with your stretches you may add some advanced moves to your schedule.

Advanced Russian Drills for Extreme Flexibility

25. The Side Stretch

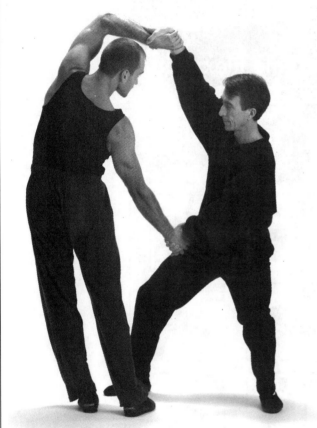

This stretch from gymnastics hits your obliques and lats hard, at the same time.

Hold on to something stationary, a training partner, a power rack, or a doorway with your hands wide apart and your body strictly sideways . Do not twist at any point!

Keep your legs straight. Push your hips away from the support

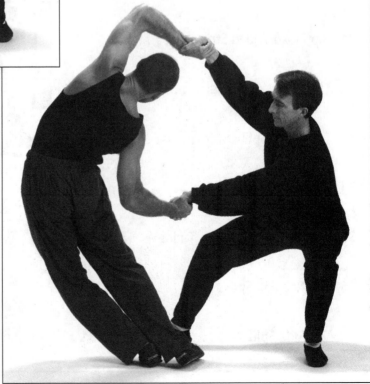

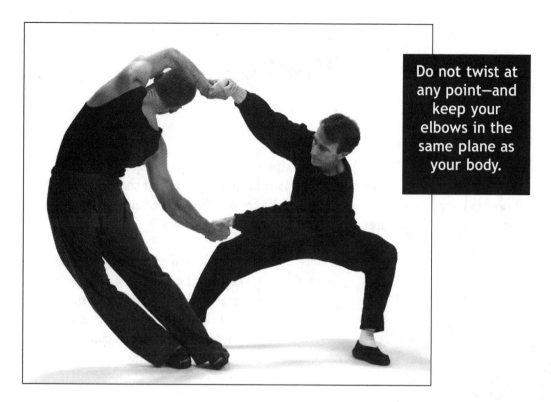

Do not twist at any point—and keep your elbows in the same plane as your body.

Inhale, contract your glutes, and pull with your top arm The elbow stays above your head!

Release and fall further away while staying in one plane.

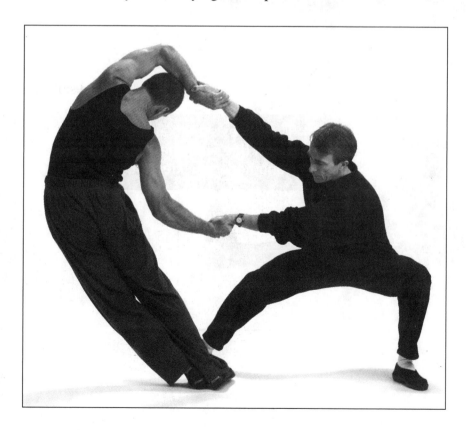

26. The Cossack

This cool stretch will loosen up your hips and improve your squatting ability. It is not nearly as tough as splits; I have placed it in the advanced section because beginners have a hard time tracking their knees properly. The knees should always be in line with the toes and never buckled in!

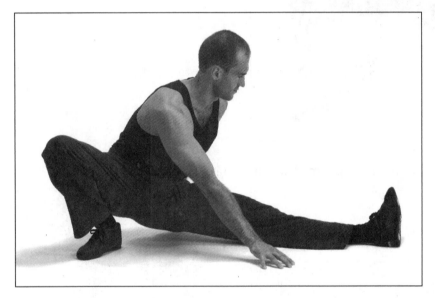

Squat down on one leg while keeping the other leg straight and relatively unloaded. You may hold on to something for balance. Squat down as deep as you can and squeeze your butt.

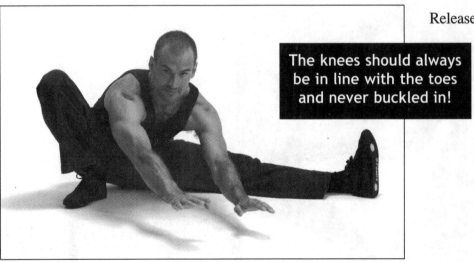

Release and sink deeper.

The knees should always be in line with the toes and never buckled in!

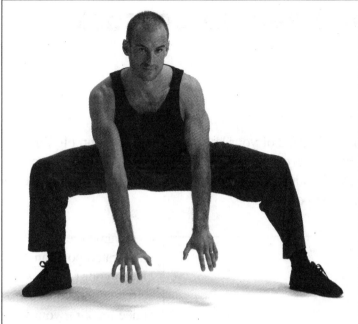

Do the drill in both directions. Change sides whenever you feel like it by pivoting near the ground.

Switch your position after each contraction to work every conceivable angle of your hip joint range of motion. Break up the distribution of weight between your feet; vary the direction where your unloaded foot is pointing; shift the weight on your support foot from your heel to your toes and back. Get a distinct feeling of 'rolling' in your hip joint when you switch positions. 'Elongating' your straight leg, as you have done during splits, will help.

Make sure to keep one leg totally straight except when you are switching sides! Understand that the Cossack stretch is not for everyone's knees.

You may combine the Cossack stretch with the Cossack mobility drill from *Super Joints*.

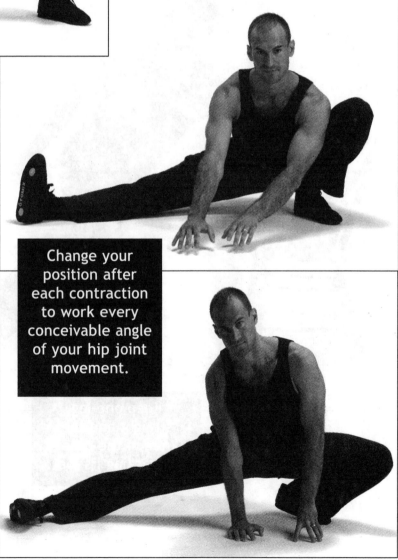

Change your position after each contraction to work every conceivable angle of your hip joint movement.

103

27. The Reverse Cossack

The so-called IT band on the outside of your knee tends to tighten up big time in runners. My buddy John Faas reports from the U.S. Navy SEAL training base in San Diego that even elite frogmen are not immune against this problem and stretch their ITs religiously. Here is the best way.

Assume the illustrated position. Keep your right leg straight and your left knee tracking your left foot for the duration.

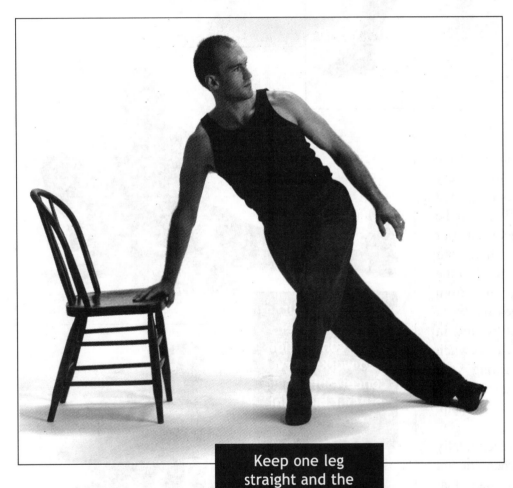

Keep one leg straight and the knee of the other leg tracking its foot.

With most of your weight on the outside of your straight right leg pivot and 'screw yourself into the ground'.

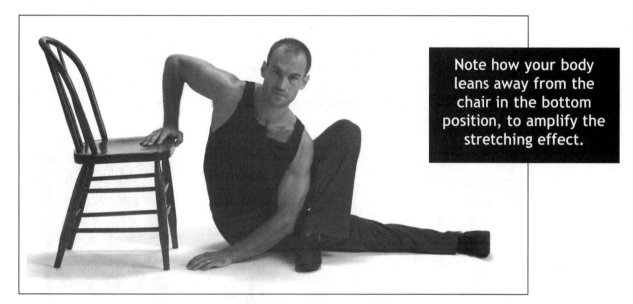

Note how your body leans away from the chair in the bottom position, to amplify the stretching effect.

Push with the outside of your right foot into the ground, then release and sink. Note how your body leans away from the chair in the bottom position to amplify the stretching effect.

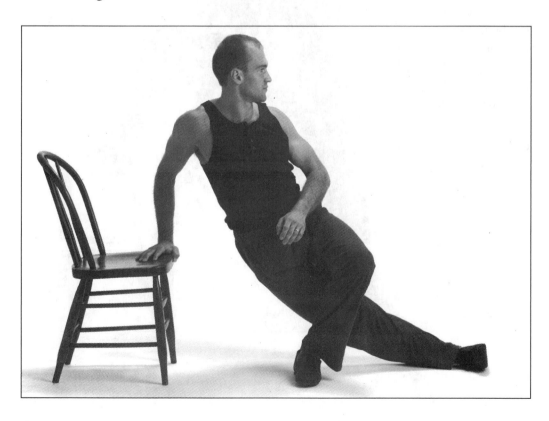

Repeat the drill with your left paw.

28. The Hip and Side Stretch

This stretch—popular in former East Germany—hits your hips in a slightly different fashion and stretches your side muscles as well. It works best if you hold a light weight; a can of mushroom soup will do for starters.

Step with one foot on a stool or another elevated surface. Do not bend your knee beyond ninety degrees throughout the stretch.

Make sure to position your floor-based leg in a manner that does not bother your knee during the stretch; the rule of thumb is to align the knee and the foot in the same direction.

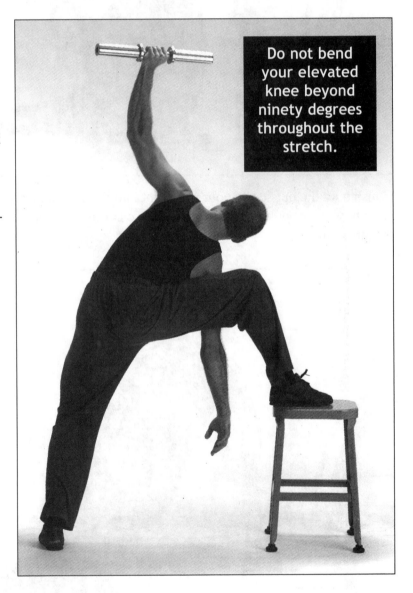

Do not bend your elevated knee beyond ninety degrees throughout the stretch.

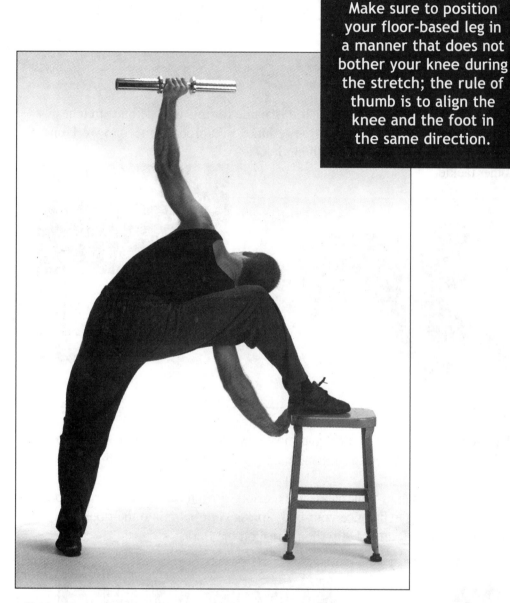

Make sure to position your floor-based leg in a manner that does not bother your knee during the stretch; the rule of thumb is to align the knee and the foot in the same direction.

Shift your weight to the heel of the elevated foot and tighten your glute. Your body will slip down inside your knee when you release the tension. The weight in your hand will help to track your body in the right groove.

If you find that you cannot keep the knee of the elevated leg out of your body's way, you need to improve your groin flexibility before having another pass at the evil GDR stretch.

29. The Crawling Lizard

'The Crawling Lizard' is a Russian folk name for this intense butt stretch. Assume the position illustrated. If you cannot, you probably need to work on your hip flexors awhile longer before giving it another tackle.

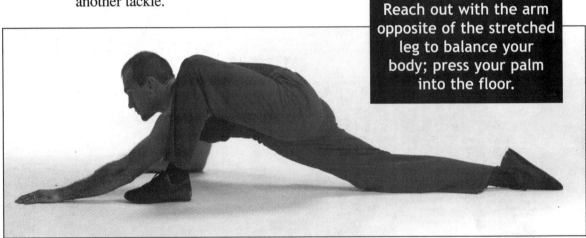

Reach out with the arm opposite of the stretched leg to balance your body; press your palm into the floor.

The front shin must be vertical and most of your weight should be on the heel of the front leg. Tighten your glutes and push your front heel through the floor.

Your body will sag as you release the tension. Reach out with the arm opposite of the stretched leg to balance your body; press your palm into the floor. Eventually your soft underbelly should rest on the floor.

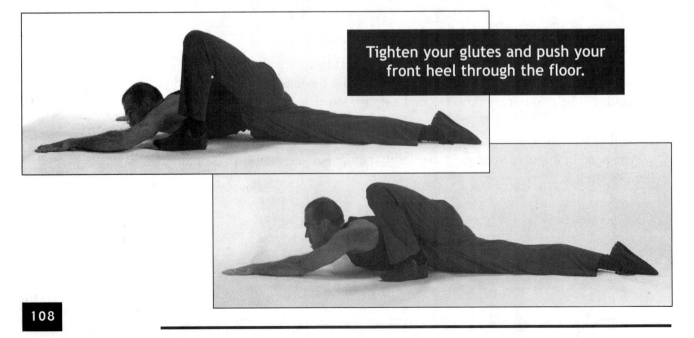

Tighten your glutes and push your front heel through the floor.

30. Hamstring Stretches

Once, thanks to good mornings, the difference has sunk in—between folding at the hip and bending from your back—you may choose from a variety of the following hamstring stretches. They all obey the same rules as the good morning: chin and chest up, back straight, dig with your heels, fold at the hip, etc. Keep your knees slightly bent or locked depending on your preference and health history. As an option, you may keep your hands behind your back to ensure a straighter spine.

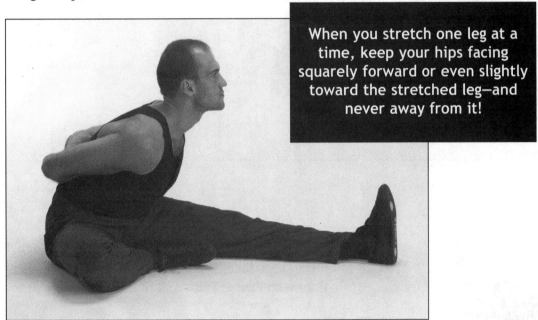

When you stretch one leg at a time, keep your hips facing squarely forward or even slightly toward the stretched leg—and never away from it!

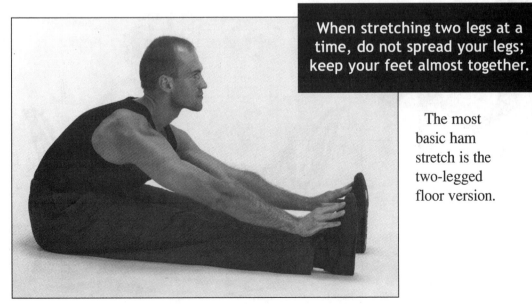

When stretching two legs at a time, do not spread your legs; keep your feet almost together.

The most basic ham stretch is the two-legged floor version.

For the one-legged version, fold one of your legs toward the opposite knee—not the other way, as in the hurtful hurdler stretch! Make sure to keep your weight over the stretched leg and not away from it!

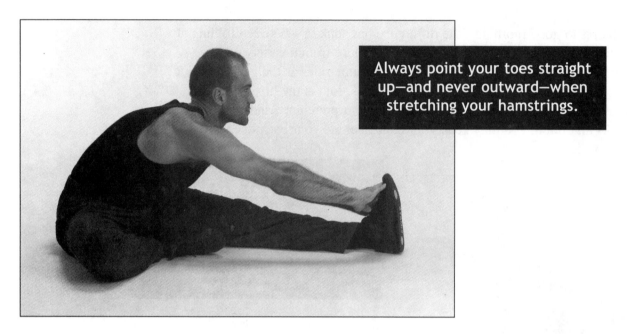

Always point your toes straight up—and never outward—when stretching your hamstrings.

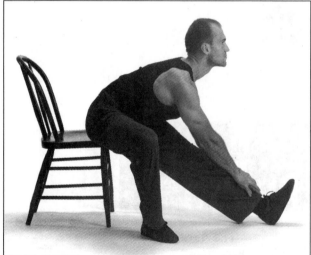

There are also easier chair versions—for the majority of Comrades who are not flexible enough just to keep their backs straight, when seated on the floor with their legs in front of them.

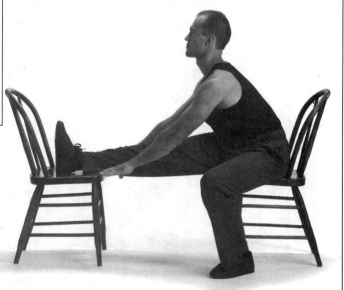

The free standing one-legged ham stretch is a good one for nearly any level. Make a point of keeping your weight over the leg you are stretching. Also, keep the bent knee of the other leg tracking your slightly turned out foot; never let your knees bow in!

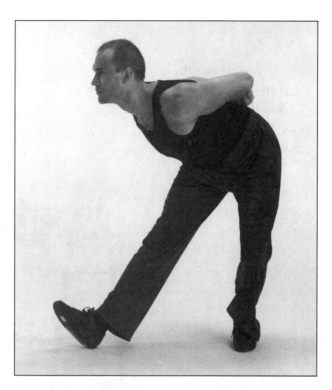

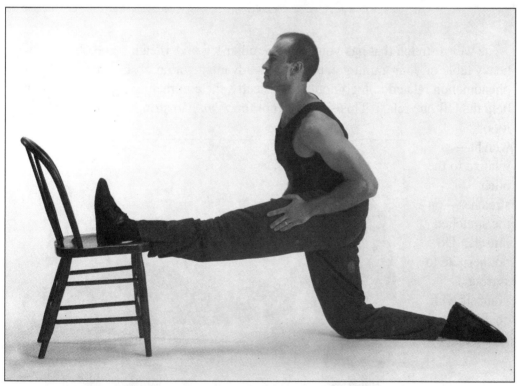

The cool knee-on-the-floor chair stretch is very user friendly, because the kneeling leg is pulling the pelvis in the right direction. Make sure to pad your knee with something soft and to watch your balance. You may surround yourself with a couple of chairs for balance if you wish.

If you choose the same stretch with your foot planted on the floor, pay attention not to wrench the knee of your support leg.

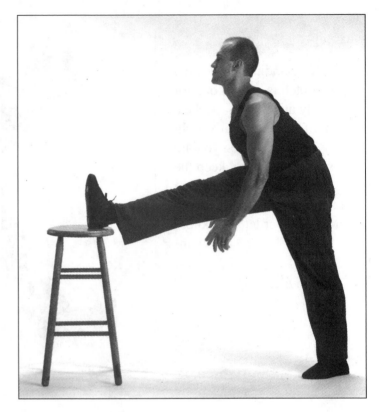

The weird stretch that has you hook the other leg underneath some object, say a heavy table or your training partner, takes advantage of an obscure neurological phenomenon related to locomotion. Basically, the contracting right hamstring will help the left one relax. This stretch is not for weak hamstrings because it places a lot of weight—relative to the other stretches—on the stretched muscle. Do not hesitate to surround yourself with chairs for safety.

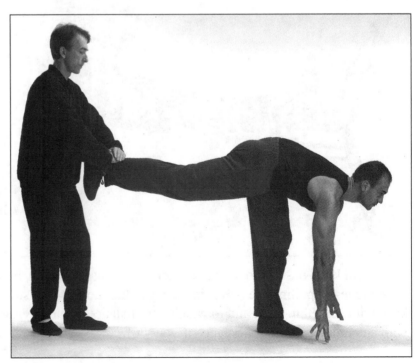

Conventional hamstring stretches encourage more flexibility in the outer hamstrings (biceps femoris) than the inner hamstrings (semimembranosus and semotendinosus). We are anything but conventional, so we shall not worry about the inner hamstrings; they will be taken care of by your groin stretches; concentrate on the outer ones. To feel more loading on the outside than the inside of the hamstring, do two things.

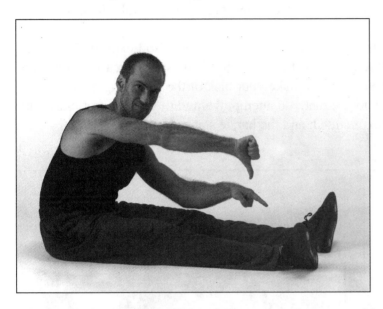

First, make a point of always pointing your toes straight up—and never outward—when stretching your hams.

Second, when you stretch one leg at a time, keep your hips facing squarely forward or even slightly toward the stretched leg—and never away from it!

31. Hip Flexor/Quad Stretches

When Comrades complain of tight quads, their problem is usually the hip flexors.

One muscle of the quadriceps group, the rectus femoris, also flexes the hip, so it has been stretched with the previous stretch. If, for some strange reason, you need to work on your knee flexion as well, take your pick of the following modified hip flexor stretches. I do not advise that you attempt them until you get proficient with the basic kneeling hip flexor stretch and the karate stance hip flexor stretch.

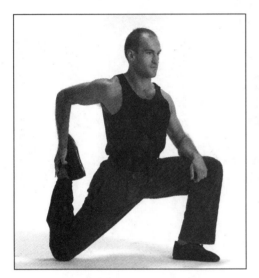

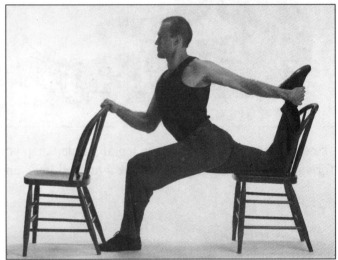

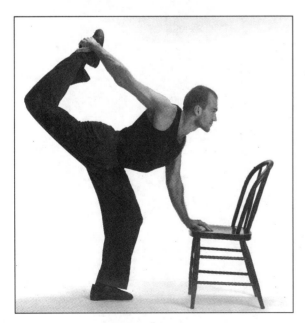

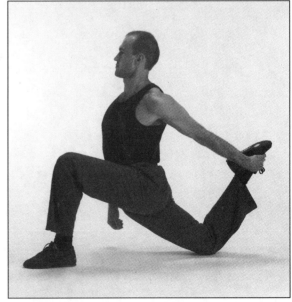

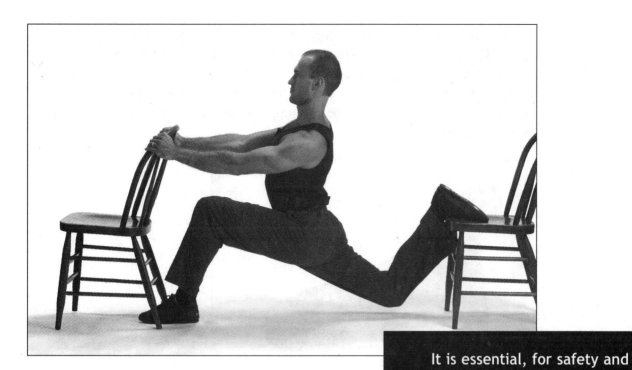

It is essential, for safety and effectiveness, to keep your hips squared off during hip flexor stretches and front splits. Contracting your glutes hard helps to align your pelvis properly.

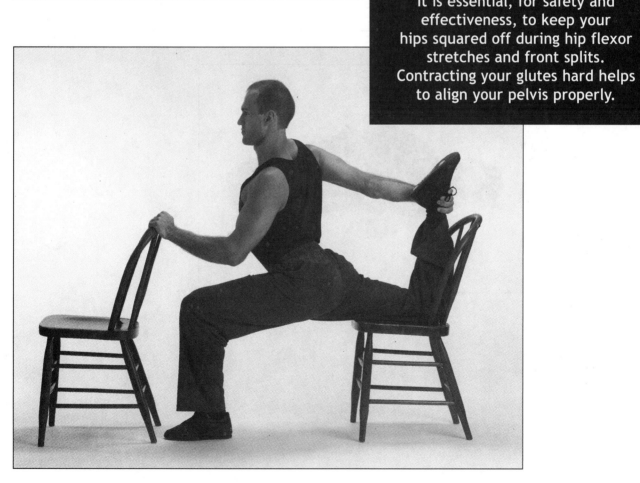

Some advanced trainees with a compelling cause may try the kneeling quad stretch. Clear it with your doctor; this stretch is way too rough on most comrades' knees! The stretch is initiated by imitating the leg extension strength exercise or trying to straighten out your legs against the floor. Be certain not to spend much time in a relaxed position when performing this stretch, to minimize the loading of the knee ligaments.

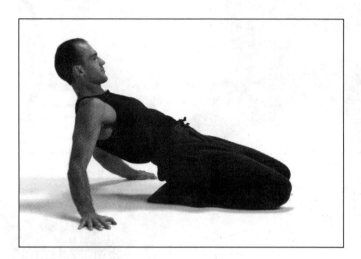

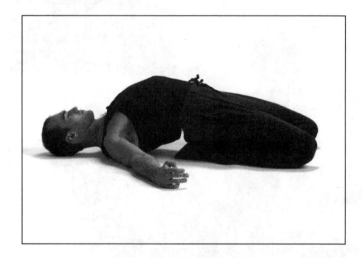

32. The Lower Calf Stretch

This stretch has found its way into the advanced section because it requires strong quads and above average body awareness. The purpose of the drill is to stretch the lower calf, or soleus, for sports and activities that require good ankle flexibility in positions with a bent knee, for example shotokan karate.

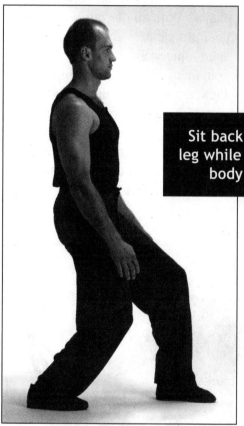

Step forward slightly with one foot while keeping the other one flat on the ground. Sit back on the rear leg while keeping your body vertical.

Sit back on the rear leg while keeping your body vertical.

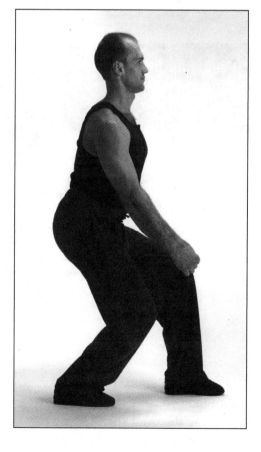

Contract your rear calf by pushing with the ball of your foot into the ground. Hold the tension—it may take a long time to tire out your calf—then release and sink straight down. Your rear knee will drop down while your heel stays on the ground.

33. The Front Split

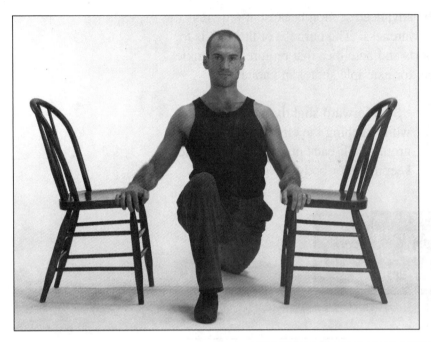

As you are working on your hip flexor and hamstring stretches, periodically test yourself on the front split. Assume the kneeling hip flexor stretch position between chairs. With all of your weight on your arms inhale and push the walls apart—the walls in front and behind you, that is. As with the hip flexor stretches, make a point of keeping your hips squared off and your rear knee facing the floor. It is a good idea to pad that knee—slip sliding magazine covers under both the knee and the feet.

Keep your hips squared off and your rear knee facing the floor.

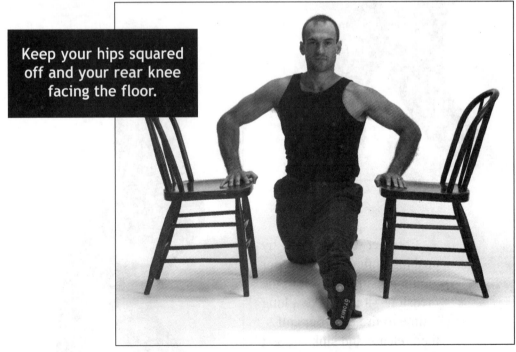

Do not force yourself down; think of making yourself longer, 'pulling your hips out of their sockets'. Once you can get within a foot of the floor, you may start practicing the front split. If you cannot, it is better to stick to your hamstring and hip flexor stretches for a while.

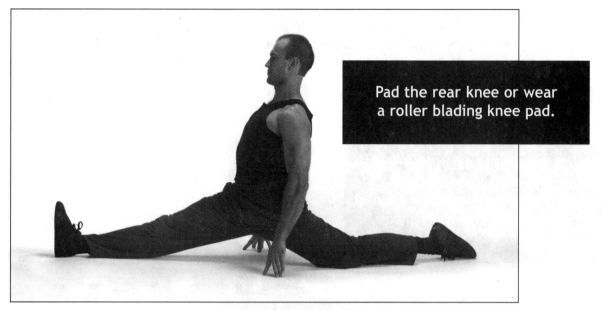

Pad the rear knee or wear a roller blading knee pad.

Carefully shift your weight away from your arms; now your hands are barely touching the chairs. Your arms are ready to catch you if you goof up somehow, but they are not carrying any weight unless your leg muscles are very weak.

Once you are very close to the floor—and you are able to rest your fists there without bending over—you may part with the chairs.

Tighten up the stretched muscles and pinch the floor. If you have a hard time doing it, just squeeze your butt and abs and everything else will follow. Do not twist your back knee! If the pressure from the floor bothers the knee—and it will, until you can get your thigh flat on the ground—pad it better. Even wear roller skating pads if you have them. This trick will help you avoid the grave mistake most splitters make—twisting your knee sideways to relieve the pressure.

Maintain steady tension in your legs, glutes, and abs. It is crucial. If you cannot put up with the progressive fatigue and pain of an extended isometric contraction, if you semi-relax your leg muscles now and then, you are wasting your time!

Hold the tension until your hamstrings and hip flexors literally collapse from exhaustion. It may take any time between a few seconds to a few minutes. It will not be enjoyable, which is irrelevant.

When you feel your tired and, perhaps, quivering, muscles involuntarily relaxing, remember the lesson of contrast breathing and let out a sigh of relief. It will help your beat-up hams and thighs go limp.

Once you have released the tension and dropped a little—just a little, to maximize safety! —catch yourself on your arms, then, with the weight on your arms, push the walls apart as you did in the beginning of the stretch. Make sure to stay upright and squared off!

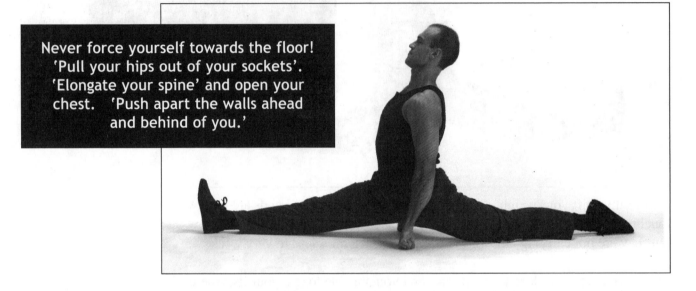

Never force yourself towards the floor! 'Pull your hips out of your sockets'. 'Elongate your spine' and open your chest. 'Push apart the walls ahead and behind of you.'

Shift your weight back to your front heel and rear knee, flex your stretched muscles, and exhaust them into submission again. Keep plugging away until you get tired, or your range of motion stops improving, whichever comes first.

Alternate the tension with the release and elongation. Eventually you will find yourself in a full split. If you do not look like the photo, if your trunk or knee is twisted and your body is leaning, you cannot claim that you can do a split!

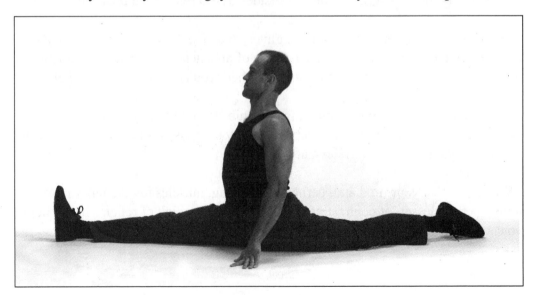

Russian specialist Fillipovich advises holding your lowest position in the splits for 10-20 sec. If you are tough, you can bump up this time to a couple of minutes and even hold the muscles under tension. Scream your heart out!

Once you are down all the way, you may increase the difficulty of the stretch by rotating your torso away from the rear leg. You could also stick some phone book sized object under your front leg.

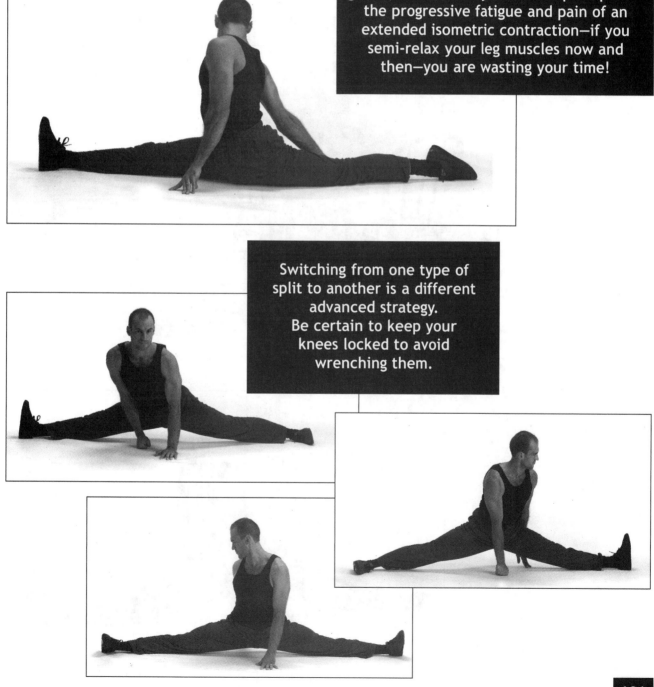

Maintain steady tension in your legs, glutes, and abs. If you cannot put up with the progressive fatigue and pain of an extended isometric contraction—if you semi-relax your leg muscles now and then—you are wasting your time!

Switching from one type of split to another is a different advanced strategy. Be certain to keep your knees locked to avoid wrenching them.

You may have noticed that when you make the transition from a side split to the front split or vice versa you end up in a 'martial arts split'. Less challenging than either the side or the front split, the martial arts split is nevertheless a good stretch. It is highly specific to karate and other kicks and may be practiced by itself, even before you are ready for the classic splits.

Starting your split workout with non-forceful split switches—they are featured in the Super Joints program as a tool for improving the mobility and health of your hip joints—is guaranteed to advance your splitting cause.

The martial arts split will not tolerate bent knees—and vice versa.

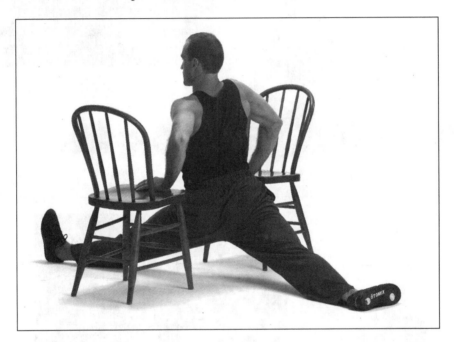

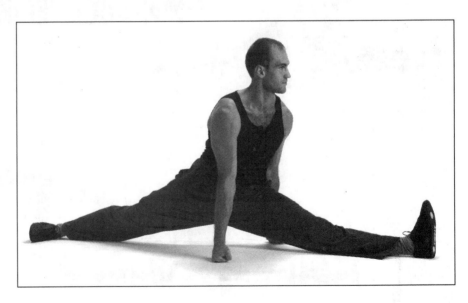

34. The Bent Press Stretch

Although this stretch looks deceptively similar to the triangle asana from yoga it has a radically different history and body mechanics. This drill is derived from the 'bent press' strength feat popularized in the XIX century by legendary Russian strongman, Eugene Sandow. The bent press stretch ranks advanced because it requires precise coordination if it is to be performed safely. Consider owning the companion videotape, to get this one right.

If you do the bent press stretch correctly you will feel it on the outside of your butt. The bent press stretch is great for 'decramping' your outer thighs after side splits and cannot be beat for relieving soreness after heavy deadlifts and squats. If you have sciatica pain from a tight piriformis muscle—not from disk problems! —ask your doctor if this stretch can fix it. This exercise's chest opening effect is nothing to sneeze at either.

Keep your chest open and your eyes on your hand or weight for the duration of the stretch.

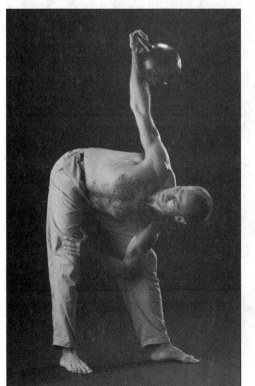

Lift your right arm overhead, eventually with a weight, and kick out your right hip to the side. The action is similar to 'crease folding' in the good morning stretch but is done more to the side than to the rear. Note the position of the feet.

Keep your right knee locked and try to keep as much weight as possible on your right leg throughout the stretch. The other knee may be bent; this is not yoga, Comrade!

Keep your chest open and your eyes on your hand or weight. Tighten up your right glutes, hold the tension for a while, then release and fold sideways. Keep your free hand wherever it is comfortable.

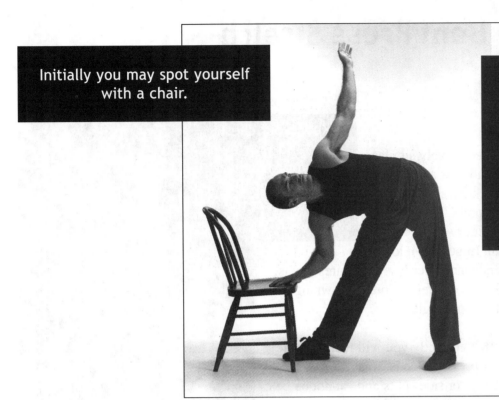

Initially you may spot yourself with a chair.

Keep the knee on the side of the elevated arm locked and try to keep as much weight as possible on this leg throughout the stretch.

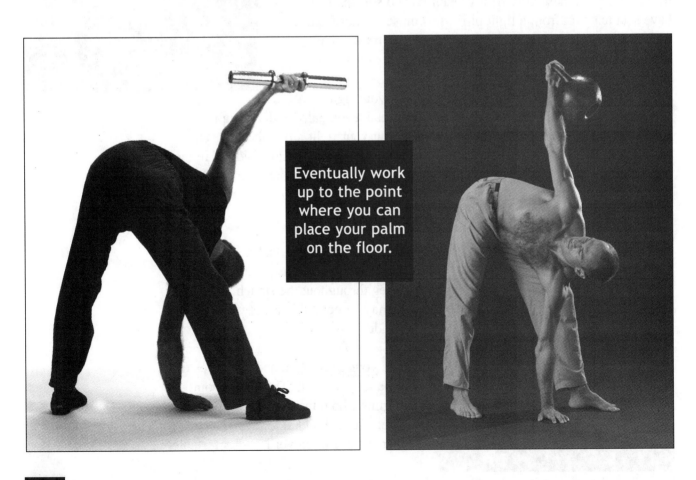

Eventually work up to the point where you can place your palm on the floor.

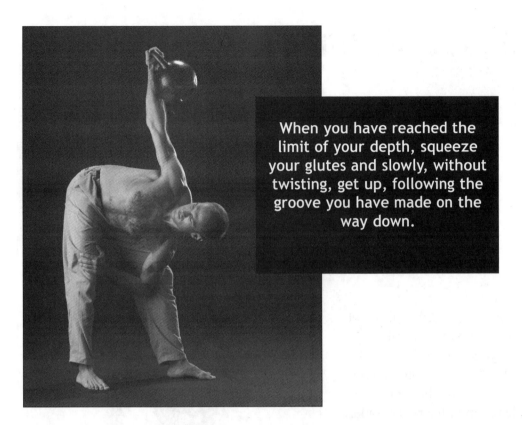

When you have reached the
limit of your depth, squeeze
your glutes and slowly, without
twisting, get up, following the
groove you have made on the
way down.

When you have reached the limit of your depth, squeeze your glutes and slowly, without twisting, get up, following the groove you have made on the way down. Naturally, work both sides.

If you like the well-rounded combination of strength, flexibility, and balance demanded by this drill, do yourself a favor and check out *The Russian Kettlebell Challenge: Xtreme Fitness for Hard Living Comrades.*

35. The Modified Reverse Triangle

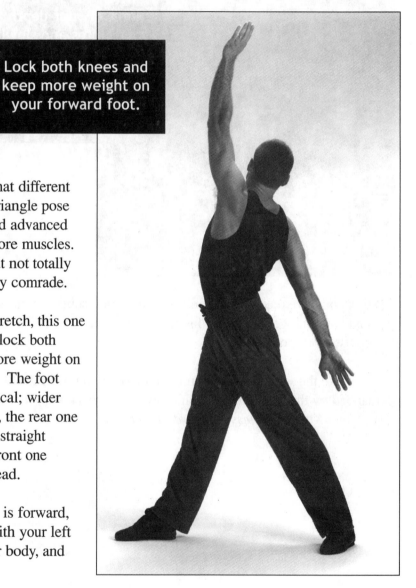

Lock both knees and keep more weight on your forward foot.

This one is not that different from the reverse triangle pose from yoga. A good advanced stretch for many core muscles. Very rewarding but not totally safe for an ordinary comrade.

Unlike the last stretch, this one demands that you lock both knees and keep more weight on your forward foot. The foot alignment is identical; wider than the shoulders, the rear one is pointing almost straight forward, and the front one almost straight ahead.

If your right foot is forward, inhale, reach up with your left arm, elongate your body, and turn to the right.

Now comes the tricky part. Fold sideways while looking up at your right hand as the left one is sliding down the right leg.

Squeeze your butt and press your hand against your leg. Relax and fold.

Carefully get up exactly as you came up. Do not forget to flex your glutes to power up your ascent.

It goes without saying, work both sides. You may use a weight but keep it light.

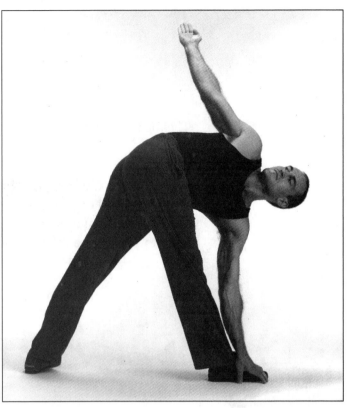

Carefully get up exactly as you came up. Do not forget to flex your glutes to power up your ascent.

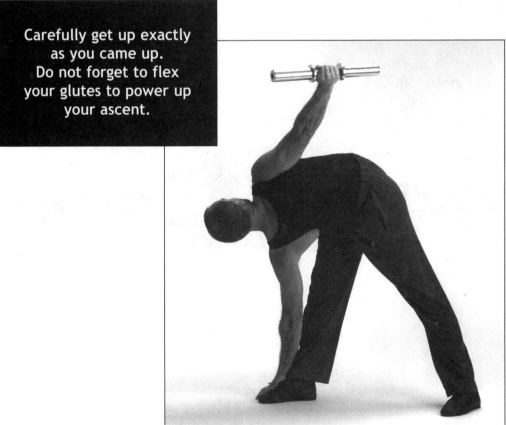

36. The Road Kill Split

The road kill stretch cannot be beat for increasing rock climbers' and dancers' turnout.

When you have achieved some proficiency in the seated groin you may ever so carefully shift all of your weight to your elbows. Your hips will be in the air and your legs will form a straight line, if viewed from above. Slowly transfer your weight to your legs and pinch the floor with your feet.

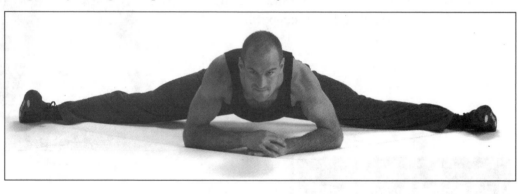

Once you have released the tension, your feet will slide apart a little. Shift your weigh to your elbows and push the walls apart even further.

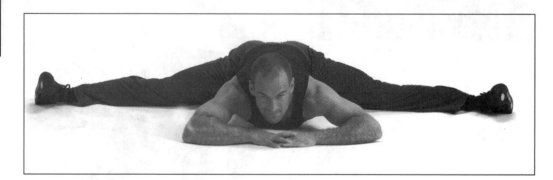

Repeat the sequence with the eventual goal of getting flatter than a roadkill!

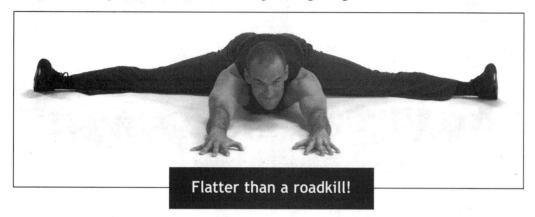

Flatter than a roadkill!

At this point you may occasionally twist your body to break things up a bit.

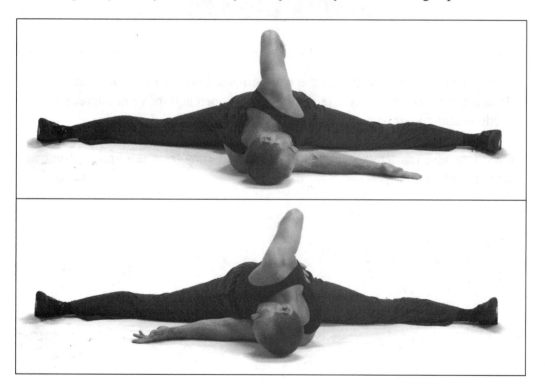

You are also are also ripe to elevate your feet for negative splits.

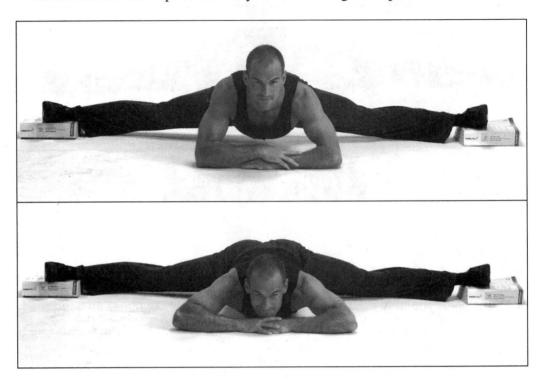

Although I use phone books on the photographs, I advise that you rig up something that does not have a tendency to split open and move in unpredictable directions under your feet. A plastic box for tools perhaps? Improvise.

Once you have mastered the road kill stretch you may try a side split. If you are tough enough, that is.

37. The Side Split

Russian commandos pride themselves on their ability to perform a 'dead split'. But, not because anyone plans on kicking the enemy in the head.

Imagine: you've ski-marched over the frozen tundra, with a hundred pounds of gear, on the wooden regulation skis known as 'coffins'. You have eaten nothing but lingonberries, dug up from under the snow. You've brushed your teeth with evergreen branches, if you are lucky enough to be that far South. Believe me, the last thing you would do is a high kick!

Anyone in his right mind sticks to the Indiana Jones school of fighting and shoots the bastards.

Even if he is out of ammo, a commando does not resort to spinning back kicks to the head. No, he'll use the dirty fighting skills of 'applied karate', of combat sambo, or the esoteric and deadly moves of Russian Martial Art. This way you get to send the bad guys to Valhalla—without wasting the energy equivalent of a Tae Bo workout, in the process.

So why bother with the side split?

Because, unless you have mastered it at the tender age of a cheerleader, the side split is one of the best exercises in mind control and pain tolerance.

Yes, the 'dead split', as the toes forward side split is called in Russia, is as painful as it looks! On one hand, pain, fear, and anxiety reduce flexibility by increasing the sensitivity of the stretch reflex. On the other hand, it is possible to will a stretch reflex not to fire! In other words, the split can be achieved, but you must go beyond good, evil, and the pain of twenty rep squats or childbirth!

Start by eating a bottle of aspirin… Just kidding. Don't be sensitive, OK? Stand on a couple of glossies and place your hands or fists on the floor in front of you. Bend forward and place your hands on the floor in front of you. I suggest that you point your fingers toward you or use your fists, but it is not a must. It also happens to be the only choice you will have in the splitting matter. Enjoy it while it lasts. You are on Soviet territory now and I am the commandant of the camp!

With your weigh on your arms, look up, open your ribcage, and push the walls apart. Keep your toes pointed more or less forward.

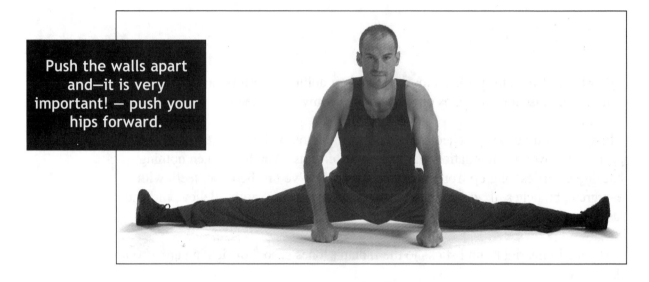

Push the walls apart and—it is very important! — push your hips forward.

Slowly transfer your weight to your legs and assume as upright a position as you can muster. Keep your lower back arched. It is a must. The pelvis usually gets in the way of your femurs when you try to spread them apart. Tilt your pelvis forward by making your lower spine go concave—and it gets out of the way!

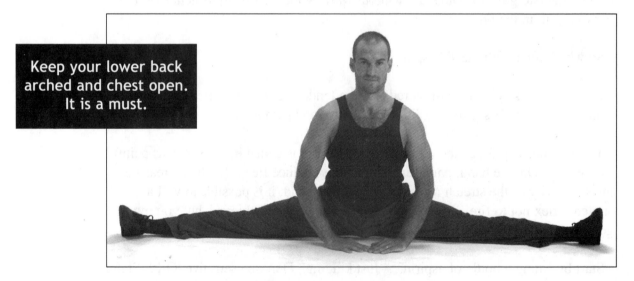

Keep your lower back arched and chest open. It is a must.

Pinch the floor with your feet with one to two thirds of your maximal strength (the stretching mode of choice is *Forced Relaxation*). Build up the tension gradually, over a couple of seconds. It is easy to get injured when you rapidly flex a stretched muscle, Comrade!

Hold steady, unwavering tension for twenty seconds, perhaps even longer, and do not forget to breathe. Although holding the contraction for such a long time is not always necessary to relax the muscle effectively, it helps to build strength.

Suddenly release the tension with a sigh of relief and allow yourself to sink a little deeper into the split. It seems impossible when your body feels like it is being torn in half, but it can be done. Relaxation is mind over matter. If you do not mind the pain, it will not matter.

Gently lift yourself up with one hand in the front and one behind you. Push the walls apart and—it is very important!—push your hips forward. Before we start hurting, you must understand that you will never, ever do a side split without positioning your pelvis in one line with your feet!

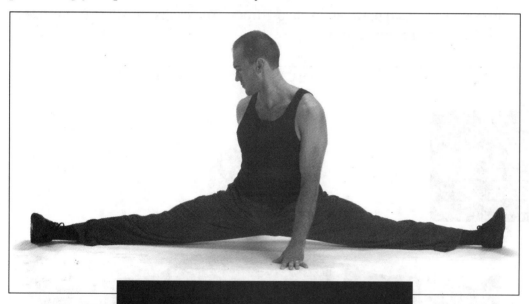

Drive your hips forward at every opportunity, try to get them in line with your feet. Push your hips forward with the help of your arms. There are three hand positions to choose from. You can push-pull with one hand in the front and one behind you; you can grip the floor in front of you with your hands and pull yourself forward; or, once you are flexible enough, you may push from behind your back.

Leaving the glutes a few inches behind the heels is a fatal mistake, which keeps many very flexible people from going down all the way in a split. They either end up falling on their butts, or sitting down on the floor with their legs spread wide, but never wide enough. This subtlety is something the devious insiders of the stretching racket would rather not reveal. The fewer people can do the splits, the more accomplished the stretch pros look.

It is your lucky day. First, I have given away the farm, and now I shall unclassify my method of mastering the proper hip alignment in the quickest possible way!

The secret to kill for is: to push your hips forward with the help of your arms.

There are three hand positions to choose from. You can push-pull with one hand in the front and one behind you...

The secret to kill for is: to push your hips forward with the help of your arms.

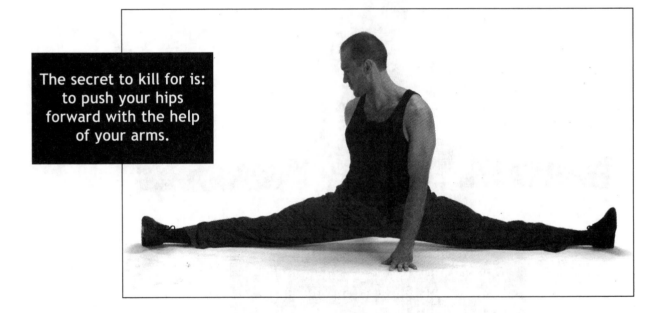

...you can grip the floor in front of you with your hands and pull yourself forward...

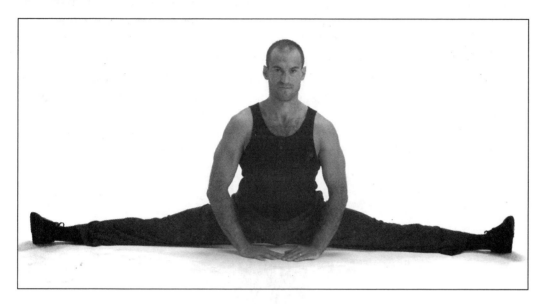

...or, once you are flexible enough, you may push from behind your back.

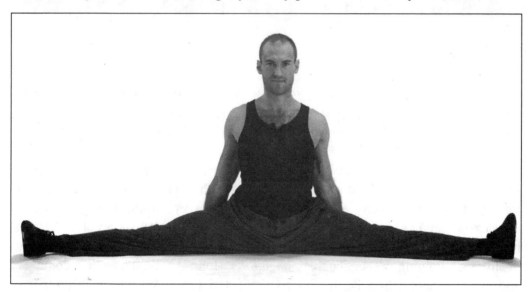

If you have diligently waited until you can do a perfect road kill split before attempting the Russian split, you will feel that the muscles in the front of your thighs resist the stretch more than your inner thighs. It is normal. It is time to shift your concentration from your groin to these front muscles: sartorius, psoas, etc. Consciously contract all of the above, the muscles underneath and in the front of your hip joints, once you have driven your hips forward.

Hold that tension! If your muscles start quivering and give out by themselves at some point during the stretch (*Clasp Knife*), do not freak and take it as a favor. As before, alternate the contractions with relaxations and the wall pressing action.

Drive your hips forward at every opportunity, and try to get them in line with your feet. If you do it right, you should be able to sit in a full split without leaning on your hands—and your legs will form a straight line when viewed from above.

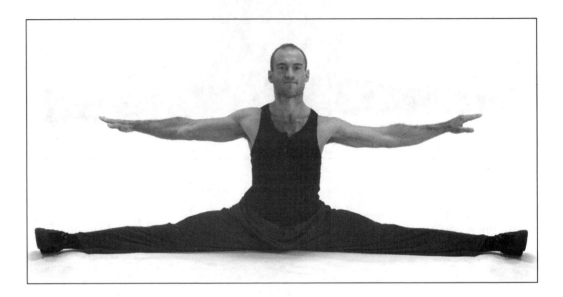

Keep at it, until you can no longer increase your stretch or you have reached your pain threshold. Carefully get out of the stretched position. Do not twist your knees and do not panic! Try to use the strength of your groin muscles to get up.

There is no way around pain if you want quick results. John Faas cannot help straining his vocal cords and soaking his T-shirt with sweat when I am putting him through the moves. Twenty-year old John is a rare exception from the generation of slackers feeling sorry for themselves. A second degree taekwondo black belt, he has been preparing for service in the SEALs since he was twelve (John is finishing his frogman training in San Diego as we speak). John is as tough as they come and still he cannot help hollering like an exorcist victim. "Are your balls on the floor yet, trooper?"—"Yes, sir!"

Although, as the U. S. Navy SEAL saying goes, "pain is just weakness leaving your body", you must differentiate between the pain of injury or overstretch and the pain of high muscular tension. The technique I am describing does not stretch your muscles but tricks them into relaxing and picks up the slack. Therefore you should feel the extreme contraction of a heavy exercise with weights, rather than the forced pull of overzealous stretching. Ease into splitting the Russian way, to learn the difference.

If pain is not a friend of yours (shame on you!), you can minimize it by emphasizing strength gains in the stretched position, over flexibility. Take your time and build up great strength at your comfortable flexibility limit, before moving deeper into the stretch. It might take you a year to work your way down into a full split, but at least you will not suffer… as much.

Split every two to three days, or as often as four times a week if you choose the 'pain light' approach. Do not do any more sets and contractions than it takes to reach your daily limit. Two to four sets work best for most people. Hold the last contraction of the last set steadily for at least thirty seconds, more if you have the fortitude.

Once you have worked your way down to the floor and want to try the suspended split a la Jean Claude Van Damme, use phone book sized plastic boxes instead of chairs. Physiologically there is no difference, but the former are less likely to put you out of commission for good.

If you hit the wall, do not ever try to excuse your lameness with your age or 'the way you are built'. Studies show that anyone with normal hip and back ROM can learn to do side splits if they learn proper alignment! Only the folks with fused vertebrae, degenerative hip joint disease, and other equally nasty problems truly cannot. The rest just do not want it bad enough. They are content to remain poorly assembled collections of body parts, devoid of any athletic ability.

How bad do YOU want it? To change your shape at will—like an advanced model quicksilver Terminator?

Most of the above stretches are demonstrated on the companion video, *Relax into Stretch.*

Relax into Stretch
delivers instant flexibility!

Conventional stretching attempts to literally elongate your tissues, which is dangerous and ineffective.

*Relax into Stretc*h simply teaches your muscles to relax into a stretch. If you compare traditional training to a messy hardware reorganization, then *Relax into Stretch* is an efficient software upgrade.

While stretching tissues may take years, changes in the nervous system are immediate! Your muscles will start noticeably elongating from your first *Relax into Stretch* practice—and within months you will have achieved a level of flexibility uncommon in our species.

Comrade,
welcome to the ranks
of mutants!
You've been Pavelized!

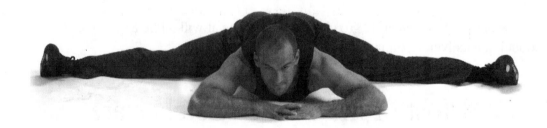

About the Author

Pavel

Pavel Tsatsouline, Master of Sports, was voted *Rolling Stone's* 'Hot Trainer' of the year in 2001. 'The Evil Russian' is the author of a number of best selling fitness books including *Super Joints* and *The Russian Kettlebell Challenge: Xtreme Fitness for Hard Living Comrades*. He is a contributing editor for Muscle Media magazine.

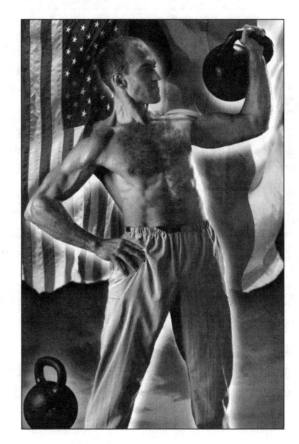

A former Soviet Special Forces instructor, Pavel was nationally ranked in the Russian ethnic sport of kettlebell lifting and holds a Soviet Physical Culture Institute degree in physiology and coaching. Tsatsouline teaches his '*low tech/high concept*' fitness approach to US military and law enforcement agencies and conducts national kettlebell instructor certification courses. Pavel has been interviewed by CNN Headline News, the Fox News Channel, USA Today, Associated Press, and EXTRA TV.

How to stay informed of the latest advances in strength and conditioning

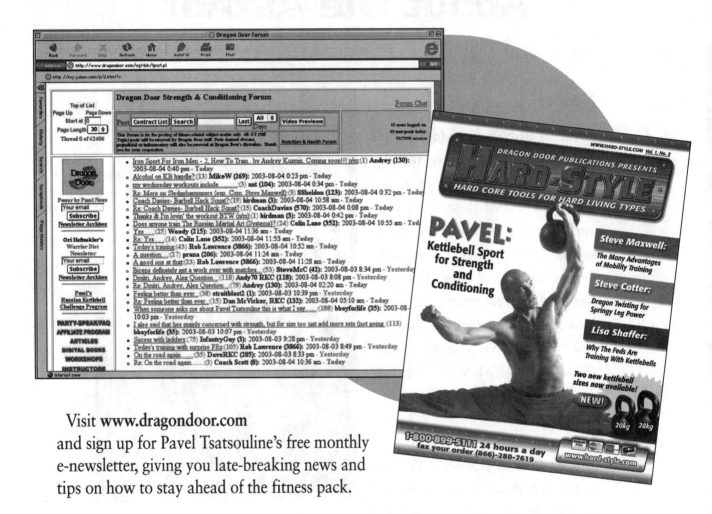

Visit **www.dragondoor.com** and sign up for Pavel Tsatsouline's free monthly e-newsletter, giving you late-breaking news and tips on how to stay ahead of the fitness pack.

Visit **http://forum.dragondoor.com/** and participate in Dragon Door's stimulating and informative **Strength and Conditioning Forum**. Post your fitness questions or comments and get quick feedback from Pavel Tsatsouline and other leading fitness experts.

Visit **www.dragondoor.com** and browse the **Articles** section and other pages for groundbreaking theories and products for improving your health and well being.

Call Dragon Door Publications at **1-800-899-5111** and request your FREE **Hard-Style** catalog of fitness books, videos, supplements and equipment.

Make it Easy on Yourself to be Flexible Fast!

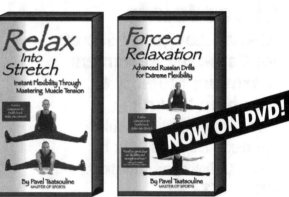

Pavel's companion videos, *Relax into Stretch* and *Forced Relaxation*, guarantee you effortlessly master every secret for super-flexibility—so you achieve the limber, stretched-out look and high performance body you always wanted.

"Pavel is the leading proponent of applied flexibility training at work in the field today. His ideas are dynamic and fresh. He shows the serious-minded fitness devotee another avenue of improvement. Real knowledge for real people interested in real progress."

—Marty Gallagher, Washington Post.com columnist, World Masters Powerlifting Champion

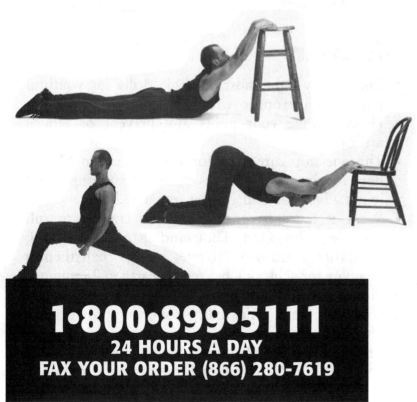

1•800•899•5111
24 HOURS A DAY
FAX YOUR ORDER (866) 280-7619

Relax into Stretch
Instant Flexibility Through Mastering Muscle Tension
By Pavel Tsatsouline
Running time: 37 minutes
Video   #V104   **$29.95**
DVD   #DV006 **$29.95**

Forced Relaxation
Advanced Russian Drills for Extreme Flexibility
By Pavel Tsatsouline
Running time: 21 minutes
Video   #V105   **$24.95**
DVD   #DV007 **$24.95**

Relax Videoor DVD Set:
Relax into Stretch &
Forced Relaxation
Video set #VS7   **$49.95**
DVD set #DVS002   **$49.95**

Relax Book and Video Set:
Relax into Stretch book and Relax into Stretch/
Forced Relaxation videos   #VBS1
$79.95

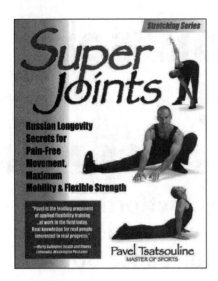

Super Joints

Russian Longevity Secrets for Pain-Free Movement, Maximum Mobility & Flexible Strength

Book By Pavel Tsatsouline
Paperback 130 pages 8.5" x 11"
Over 100 photos and illustrations
#B16 $34.95

Super Joints

Video and DVD

With Pavel Tsatsouline
Running Time 33 minutes
Video **#V108 $24.95**
DVD **#DV003 $24.95**

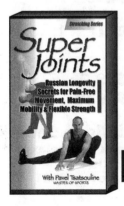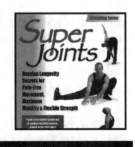

"The Do-It-Now, Fast-Start, Get-Up-and-Go, Jump-into-Action Bible for HIGH PERFORMANCE and LONGER LIFE"

You have a choice in life. You can sputter and stumble and creak your way along in a process of painful, slow decline—or you can take charge of your health and become a human dynamo.

And there is no better way to insure a long, pain-free life than performing the right daily combination of joint mobility and strength-flexibility exercises.

In *Super Joints*, Russian fitness expert Pavel Tsatsouline shows you exactly how to quickly achieve and maintain peak joint health—and then use it to improve every aspect of your physical performance.

Only the foolish would deliberately ignore the life-saving and life-enhancing advice Pavel offers in *Super Joints*. Why would anyone willingly subject themselves to a life of increasing pain, degeneration and decrepitude? But for an athlete, a dancer, a martial artist or any serious performer, *Super Joints* could spell the difference between greatness and mediocrity.

Discover:

* The twenty-eight most valuable drills for youthful joints and a stronger stretch
* How to save your joints and prevent or reduce arthritis
* The one-stop care-shop for your inner Tin Man—how to give your nervous system a tune up, your joints a lube-job and your energy a recharge
* What it takes to go from cruise control to full throttle: The One Thousand Moves Morning Recharge Amosov's "bigger bang" calisthenics complex for achieving heaven-on earth in 25 minutes
* How to make your body feel better than you can remember—active flexibility fosporting prowess and fewer injuries
* The amazing Pink Panther technique that may add a couple of feet to your stretch the first time you do it

"Injuries Flee the Scene of the Crime, Rehab Miracles Become Norm—Using *Super Joints* Fast Response, Rescue-Your-Own-Body, Super-Relief Program"

"Three days after I initially fractured my elbow I started doing *Super Joints* and within two weeks I had full mobility back in my right arm. I was supposed to attend Occupational Therapy, but when I got there they were so shocked and amazed at my progress that they sent me home. I guess they've never seen someone regain their mobility so fast."—Tonya Ehlebracht, US Army

"*Super Joints* is excellent. It is also saving me a good deal of money. I've had to lay off of heavy squatting and deadlifting because of a back injury. My active release therapist/chiro is amazed at how quickly I am making progress—my alignment doesn't return to crap after an adjustment. I credit the progress mainly to Super Joints." From: chris m., 2003-05-18

"I am 58 and need to keep my joints oiled. I have had very good results with *Super Joints* My knees and elbows don't ache anymore." From: seeahill, 2002-11-07

"I already feel "younger." I'm also noticing an ability to better withstand rolling in Jiu Jitsu class—I don't have to tap quite as often, even in bad positions. Super Joints is a fantastic, fantastic book. I think that everyone should do *Super Joints*." From: **Dan McVicker, RKC**, 2003-05-18

"As the owner of a sixty-four year old body and as the practitioner of a sedentary job, I have lost some range of motion. The movements in this book have helped me in several ways: 1) Improved the range of rotation of my head. 2) Improved the movement and reduced the pain in the right shoulder injured several years ago. 3) Helped alleviate tension in the neck and traps where I tend to carry stress. 4) Improved my posture helping me look less like a wizened old man."—**Comrade Floyd, Amazon.com**

"*Super Joints* = Super ROM. Get the book and you'll realize what you've been missing by just stretching. It's more about maintaining the youthful fluidity of the joints which is lost through age and or abuse." From: Larry Dibble, 2002-05-09

Look at all you get to live longer and feel better with *SUPER JOINTS:*

Foreword

Who needs *Super Joints?*...the needs-based survey for super-healthy joint owners...decreasing the odds of injuries...how to develop the right blend of strength and flexibility and improve your survival odds...for better performance...*active flexibility* versus *passive flexibility*...restoring youthful mobility...flexibility development for young athletes...improving posture...kicking-range...improving passive flexibility.

Part One: Joint Health and Mobility

How to keep your one hundred joints running smooth...how *Mobility Drills* can save your joints and prevent or reduce arthritis ...the *theory of limit loads*...Amosov's daily complex of joint mobility exercises...Lying Behind-the-Head Leg Raises...Standing Toe-Touch...Arm Circles... Side bends... Shoulder Blade Reach...Torso Turn...Knee Raises...Pushups...Roman Chair Situps...how to make the Roman chair situp safer...*paradoxical breathing*...squats... the secrets of safer back bending... Amosov's vital tip for creating a surge in your fountain-of-youth calisthenics.

The distinct difference between *joint mobility* and *muscle flexibility* training...Amosov's "three stages of joint health"...appropriate maintenance/prevention strategies for the three stages...how to get started and how to ramp up....the correct tempos for best results—Amosov's way and Pavel's way...when best to perform your mobility drills... shakin' up your proprioceptors—the one-stop care-shop for your inner Tin Man...how to give your nervous system a tune up, your joints a lube-job and your energy a recharge.

From cruise control to full throttle: *The One Thousand Moves Morning Recharge*—Academician Amosov's "bigger bang" calisthenics complex—how to add more cardio and more strengthening to you joint mobility program...adding One Legged Jumps, Stomach Sucks and *The Birch Tree*—how to achieve heaven-on-earth in 25-40 minutes.

Checking yourself...are your joints mobile enough?—F. L. Dolenko's battery of joint mobility tests...four tests for the cervical spine...two for the thoracic and lumbar spine...four for the shoulder girdle...two for the elbows...three for the wrists...three for the hips...and two for the knee joints.

The Drills: Joint Mobility

Illustrated descriptions and special tips:
Three plane neck movements—deceptively simple but great for bad necks...*Shoulder circles*...*Fist exercise*...*Wrist rotations*...*Elbow circles*...how to avoid contracture or age-related shortening...*The Egyptian*—an awesome shoulder loosener popular with Russian martial artists... *Russian Pool*—for super-cranking your shoulders...*Arm circles*—for all the ROM your shoulders need......*Ankle circles*...*Knee circles*...*Squats*...finding the sweet spot...why deep squats are essential and how to avoid injury with correct performance...*Hula hoop*— a favorite of Russian Phys. Ed. Teachers, good for your

lower back and hips...*Belly dance*—a must for martial artists...*The Cossack*—a great drill for the hip joints and your quest for splits...what *never* to do with your knees...*Split switches*—an excellent adjunct to your *Relax into Stretch* split training and simply dandy for your hips...*Spine flexion/extension*...why spine decompression is vital to spine health and mobility...*Spine rotation*...mobility drills for your spine as a top priority for rejuvenation.

Part Two: Strength-Flexibility Plus More Joint Mobility

How to make your body feel better than you can remember...active flexibility for sporting prowess and fewer injuries...*agonists* and *antagonists*...basic active flexibility training...how long to hold an active stretch...how to "Reach the Mark" —using the *ideomotor effect* to successfully extend your stretch... how strength coach Bill Starr develops active and passive flexibility.

How to perform the *'Pink Panther'* technique...taking advantage of the *Ukhtomsky reflex*...how one physical therapist used the Pink Panther to add a couple of feet to her hamstring stretch in one set...the partner hamstring stretch.

Is active isolated stretching any good?—the bottom line on AIS...the demographics of stretching...how and why your age and sex should dictate your choice of stretching exercises...the best techniques for young girls and boys—and what to avoid...a special warning for pregnant women...what adults should do...the elderly...and adolescents.

Stretching to help slumped shoulders...*stretch weakness* and *tight weakness*...how to address the weakness of the overstretched muscles and the tightness of their antagonists...two respected Russian regimens for better posture...understanding the vital difference between a tight and a toned muscle...the *Davis Law*...functional and dysfunctional tension.

The Drills: Strength-Flexibility Plus More Joint Mobility

Illustrated descriptions and special tips:
Windmill—for effectively improving the spine's rotation...*Pink Panther straight-legged situp*—the drill that can add a palm's length to your toe touch in minutes...*Bridge*—awesome for opening up the chest and improving spine extension...some warnings for those with back and wrists problems...how to dramatically improve your bridges with the *Relax into Stretch* hip flexor stretches.

'Bathtub push'—opens up the chest, great for posture and a must for a big bench press...how to develop an actively flexible spine with minimal disc loading—three tips from Russian experts...*'Ghost Pulling Knife'*—great for correcting "computer hunch"... *Shoulder dislocate with a bungee cord*—the Olympic weightlifter favorite for mutant shoulder flexibility...*Shoulder blade spread*—a popular stretch among old time strong men...*Side wall reach...Pink Panther knee chambers and kicks*—to dramatically improve the height and precision of your kicks...a S.W.A.T. team favorite... a unique stretching technique for high kicks from the Russian army's top hand-to-hand combat instructor...*Pink Panther arabesque*...add more height and power to your kicks with the *'Scissors maneuver'*.

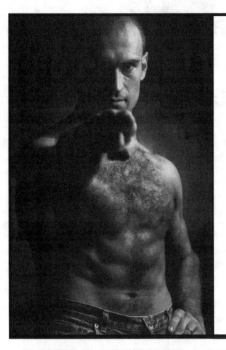
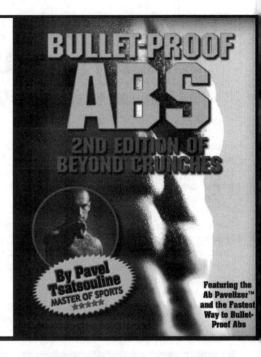

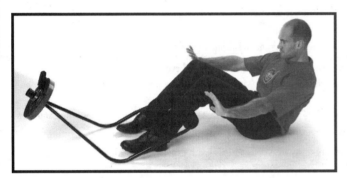
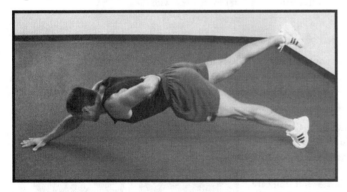
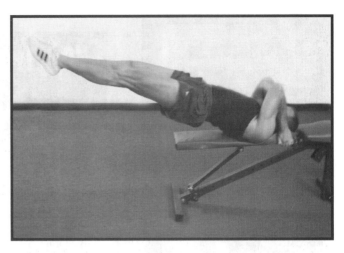
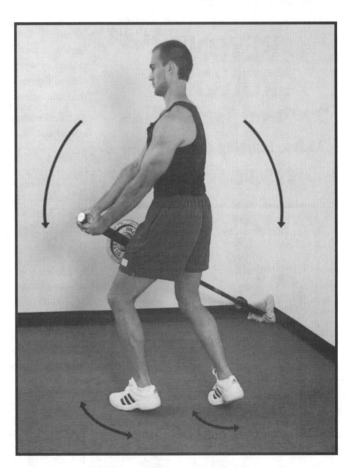

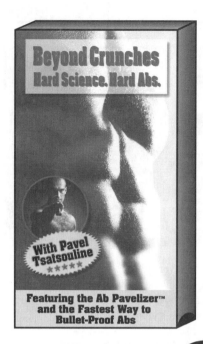

Beyond Crunches
Hard Science. Hard Abs.

With Pavel Tsatsouline
★★★★★

Featuring the Ab Pavelizer™ and the Fastest Way to Bullet-Proof Abs

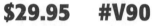
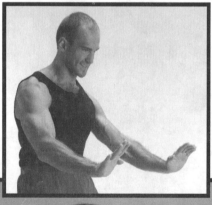
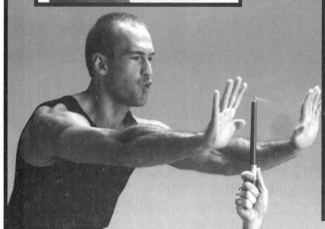
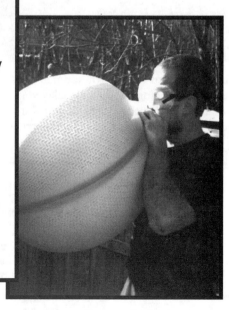

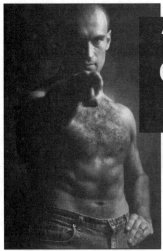

"New Ab Machine Exposes Frauds, Fakes and Cheaters–But Rewards Faithful with the Most Spectacular Abs This Side of Heaven"

The Ab Pavelizer™ II
Item # P12

$139.95

10-25 lb Olympic plate required for correct use.
(You will need to supply your own plate)

#P12

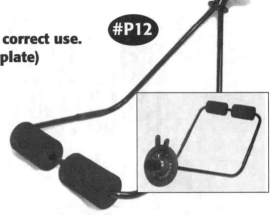

You know, it's a crying shame to cheat on your abs. Your abs are your very core, your center. Your abs define you, man or woman. So why betray them with neglect and less-than-honest carryings-on? That's bad! And everybody always knows! Rationalize all you want, hide all you want, but weak, flabby abs scream your lack of self-respect to all comers. Why live at all, if you can't hold your head up high and own a flat stomach?

Fortunately, you can now come clean, get honest and give your abs the most challenging, yet rewarding workout of their lives. And believe me, they will love you for ever!

Maybe you've been misled. Maybe you think you have to flog out hundreds of situps to get spectacular abs? Ho! Sorry, **but with abs, repetition is the mother of insanity.** Forget about it! You're just wasting your time! You're just fooling around! No wonder you're still not satisfied!

No, if you <u>really, really</u> want abs-to-die-for then: INTENSITY IS EVERYTHING!

And here lies the secret of **The Ab Pavelizer™ II**. It's all

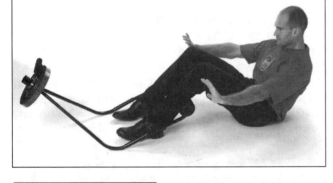

FREE BONUS:

Comes with a four page detailed instruction guide on how to use and get the most out of your Ab Pavelizer™ II. Includes two incredible methods for massively intensifying your ab workout with *Power* and *Paradox Breathing*.

in the extreme, unavoidable intensity it thrusts on you. No room for skulkers or shirkers. No room at all! Either get with the program or slink back under the stone from under which you crept.

You see, The Ab Pavelizer™ II's new sleek-'n-light design guarantees a perfect sit-up by forcing you to do it right. Now, escape or half-measures are impossible. Sit down at the Ab Pavelizer™ II and a divine slab of abs will be served up whether you like it or not. You'll startle yourself in your own mirror!

The secret to the Ab Pavelizer™ II is in the extra-active resistance it provides you. The cunning device literally pushes up against your calves (you'd almost swear it was a cruel, human partner) and forces you to recruit your glutes and hamstrings.

Two wonderful and amazing things happen.

First, it is virtually impossible to do the Janda situp wrong unless you start with a jerk. Second, the exercise becomes MUCH harder than on the Ab Pavelizer™ Classic. And "Much Harder" is Russian for "Quicker Results."

It is astonishingly hard to sit up all the way when the new Ab Pavelizer™ II is loaded with enough weight, 10-35 pounds for most comrades. If you can do three sets of five reps you will already have awesome abs.

A Great Added Benefit: Are you living in an already over-cluttered space? Want to conveniently hide the secret of your abs-success from envious neighbors? The new Ab Pavelizer™ II easily and quickly folds away in a closet or under your bed. Once prying eyes have left, you can put it up again in seconds for another handshake with heaven—or hell, depending on your perspective.

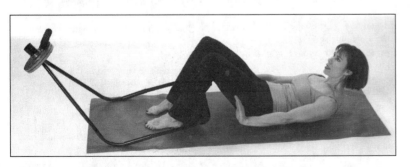

1•800•899•5111 24 HOURS A DAY, OR FAX: (866) 280-7619

Look WAY YOUNGER than Your Age
Have a LEAN, GRACEFUL, Athletic-Looking Body
Feel AMAZING, Feel VIGOROUS, Feel BEAUTIFUL
Have MORE Energy and MORE Strength to
Get MORE Done in Your Day

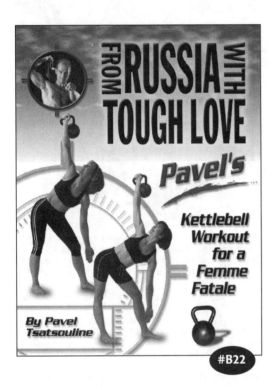

From Russia with Tough Love
Pavel's Kettlebell Workout for a Femme Fatale
Book   By Pavel Tsatsouline
Paperback   184 pages   8.5" x 11"
#B22 $34.95

In Russia, kettlebells have long been revered as the fitness-tool of choice for Olympic athletes, elite special forces and martial artists. The kettlebell's ballistic movement challenges the body to achieve an unparalleled level of physical conditioning and overall strength.

But until now, the astonishing benefits of the Russian kettlebell have been unavailable to all but a few women. Kettlebells have mostly been the sacred preserve of the male professional athlete, the military and other hardcore types. That's about to change, as Russian fitness expert and best selling author PAVEL, delivers the first-ever kettlebell program for women.

It's wild, but women really CAN have it all when they access the magical power of Russian kettlebells. Pavel's uncompromising workouts give *across-the-board, simultaneous, spectacular and immediate results* for all aspects of physical fitness: strength, speed, endurance, fat-burning, you name it. Kettlebells deliver any and everything a woman could want—if she wants to be in the best-shape-ever of her life.

And one handy, super-simple tool—finally available in woman-friendly sizes—does it all. No bulky, expensive machines. No complicated gizmos. No time-devouring trips to the gym.

Into sports? Jump higher. Leap further. Kick faster. Hit harder. Throw harder. Run with newfound speed. Swim with greater power. Endure longer. Wow!

Working hard?   Handle stress with ridiculous ease. Blaze thru tasks in half the time. Radiate confidence. Knock 'em dead with your energy and enthusiasm.

Can't keep up with your kids? Not any more! They won't know what hit them.

Just wanna have fun? Feel super-relaxed from the endorphin-rush of your life, dance all night and feel finer-than-fine the next morning…and the next…and the next.

Got attitude?   Huh! Then try Pavel's patented Russian Kettlebell workouts. Now, THAT'S attitude!

Just some of what From Russia with Tough Love reveals:

- How the *Snatch* eliminates cellulite, firms your butt, and gives you the cardio-ride of a lifetime
- How to get as strong as you want, without bulking up
- How the *Swing* melts your fat and blasts your hips 'n thighs
- How to supercharge your heart and lungs without aerobics
- How to shrink your waist with the *Power Breathing Crunch*
- How the *Deck Squat* makes you super flexible
- An incredible exercise to tone your arms and shoulders

- The *Clean-and-Press*—for a magnificent upper body
- *The real secret to great muscle tone*
- The *Overhead Squat* for explosive leg strength
- How to *think* yourself stronger—yes, really!
- The queen of situps—for those who can hack it
- Cool combination exercises that deliver an unbelievable muscular and cardiovascular workout in zero time
- An unreal drill for a powerful and flexible waist, back, and hips
- How to perform multiple mini-sessions for fast-lane fitness

"Download this tape into your eager cells and watch in stunned disbelief as your body reconstitutes itself, almost overnight"

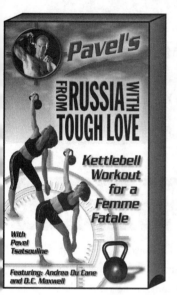

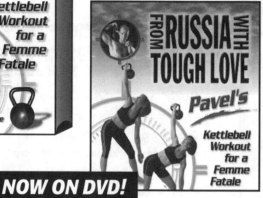

NOW ON DVD!

From Russia with Tough Love
Pavel's Kettlebell Workout for a Femme Fatale
With Pavel Tsatsouline
Running Time: 1hr 12 minutes
VIDEO **#V110** **$29.95**   DVD **#DV002** **$29.95**

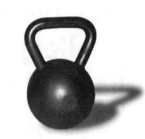

The Sure-Fire Secret to Looking Younger, Leaner and Stronger <u>AND</u> Having More Energy to Get a Whole Lot More Done in the Day

---

What you'll discover when "Tough" explodes on your monitor:

- The *Snatch*—to eliminate cellulite, firm your butt, and give you the cardio-workout of a lifetime
- The *Swing*— to fry your fat and slenderize hips 'n thighs
- The *Power Breathing Crunch*—.to shrink your waist
- The *Deck Squat*— for strength and super-flexiblity
- An incredible exercise to tone your arms and shoulders
- The *Clean-and-Press*— for a magnificent upper body
- The *Overhead Squat*— for explosive leg strength
- The queen of situps— for a flat, flat stomach
- Combination exercises that wallop you with an unbelievable muscular and cardio workout

---

Spanking graphics, a kick-ass opening, smooth-as-silk camera work, Pavel at his absolute dynamic best, two awesome femme fatales, and a slew of fantastic KB exercises, many of which were not included on the original Russian Kettlebell Challenge video.

At one hour and twenty minutes of rock-solid, cutting-edge information, this video is value-beyond-belief. I challenge any woman worth her salt not to be able to completely transform herself physically with this one tape.

"In six weeks of kettlebell work, I lost an inch off my waist and dropped my heart rate 6 beats per minute, while staying the same weight. I was already working out when I started using kettlebells, so I'm not a novice. There are few ways to lose fat, gain muscle, and improve your cardio fitness all at the same time; I've never seen a better one than this."
—*Steven Justus, Westminster, CO*

"Kettlebells are without a doubt the most effective strength/endurance conditioning tool out there. I wish I had known about them 15 years ago!"
—*Santiago, Orlando, FL*

"I have practiced Kettlebell training for a year and a half. I now have an anatomy chart back and have gotten MUCH stronger."
—*Samantha Mendelson, Coral Gables, FL*

"I know now that I will never walk into a gym again - who would? It is absolutely amazing how much individual accomplishment can be attained using a kettlebell. Simply fantastic. I would recommend it to anyone at any fitness level, in any sport."
—*William Hevener, North Cape May, NJ*

"It is the most effective training tool I have ever used. I have increased both my speed and endurance, with extra power to boot. It wasn't even a priority, but I lost some bodyfat, which was nice. However, increased athletic performance was my main goal, and this is where the program really shines."
—*Tyler Hass, Walla Walla, WA*

If you are looking for a
SUPREME EDGE
in your chosen sport —seek no more!

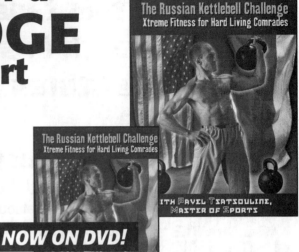

NOW ON DVD!

The Russian Kettlebell Challenge–Xtreme Fitness for Hard Living Comrades

Book By Pavel Tsatsouline
Paperback 170 pages

#B15 $34.95

With Pavel Tsatsouline
Running Time: 32 minutes

Video #V103 $39.95
DVD   #DV001 $39.95

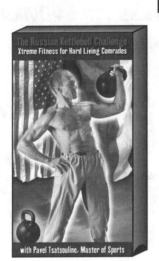

Both the Soviet Special Forces and numerous world-champion Soviet Olympic athletes used the ancient Russian Kettlebells as their secret weapon for xtreme fitness. Thanks to the kettlebell's astonishing ability to turbocharge physical performance, these Soviet supermen creamed their opponents time-and-time again, with inhuman displays of raw power and explosive strength.

Now, former Spetznaz trainer, international fitness author and nationally-ranked kettlebell lifter, Pavel Tsatsouline, delivers this secret Soviet weapon into your own hands. You NEVER have to be second best again! Here is the first-ever complete kettlebell training program—for Western shock-attack athletes who refuse to be denied—and who'd rather be dead than number two.

- **Get really, really nasty—with a commando's wiry strength, the explosive agility of a tiger and the stamina of a world-class ironman**
- **Own the single best conditioning tool for killer sports like kickboxing, wrestling, and football**
- **Watch in amazement as high-rep kettlebells let you hack the fat off your meat—without the dishonor of aerobics and dieting**
- **Kick your fighting system into warp speed—with high-rep snatches and clean-and-jerks**

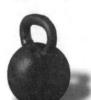

  - **Develop steel tendons and ligaments—with a whiplash power to match**
  - **Effortlessly absorb ballistic shocks—and laugh as you shrug off the hardest hits your opponent can muster**
  - **Go ape on your enemies—with gorilla shoulders and tree-swinging traps**

PRAISE FOR *THE RUSSIAN KETTLEBELL CHALLENGE*

"In *The Russian Kettlebell Challenge*, Pavel Tsatsouline presents a masterful treatise on a superb old-time training tool and the unique exercises that yielded true strength and endurance to the rugged pioneers of the iron game. Proven infinitely more efficient than any fancy modern exercise apparatus, the kettlebell via Pavel's recommendations is adaptable to numerous high and low rep schemes to offer any strength athlete, bodybuilder, martial artist, or sports competitor a superior training regimen. As a former International General Secretary of the International All-Round Weightlifting Association, I not only urge all athletes to study Mr. Tsatsouline's book and try these wonderful all-round kettlebell movements, but plan to recommend that many kettlebell lifts again become part of our competitions!"—**John McKean,** current IAWA world and national middleweight champion

"Kettlebells are unsurpassed as a medium for increasing strength and explosive power. Thanks to Pavel Tsatsouline, I have now rewritten my training program to include kettlebell training, for athletes of all disciplines from Professional Football to Olympic sprinters."—**Coach John Davies**

"Everybody with an interest in the serious matter of body regulation over a lifetime should commit themselves to Pavel's genre of knowledge and his distinct techniques of writing. Any one of the dozens of suggestions you hit upon will pay for the *Russian Kettlebell Challenge* hundreds of times."—**Len Schwartz,** author of *Heavyhands: the Ultimate Exercise System* and *The Heavyhands Walking Book!*

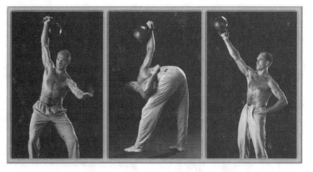
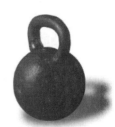
SECTION ONE
The History of the Russian Kettlebell—How and Why a Low-Tech Ball of Iron Became the National Choice for Super-Tech Results

Vodka, pickle juice, kettlebell lifting, and other Russian pastimes

'The working class sport'

Finally: Xtreme all around fitness!
Why Soviet science considers kettlebells to be one of the best tools for all around physical development....

Kettlebells in the Red Army
The Red Army catches on....every Russian military unit equipped with K-bells....the perfect physical conditioning for military personnel....the vital combination of strength and endurance....*Girevoy sport* delivers unparalleled cardio benefits....why *Spetznaz* personnel owe much of their wiry strength, explosive agility, and stamina to kettlebells....

SECTION TWO
Special Applications—How The Russian Kettlebell Can Dramatically Enhance Your Chosen Endeavor

Kettlebells for combat sports
Russian wrestlers do lion's share of conditioning with kettlebells.... Why KB one arm snatches work better than Hindu squats....KB's strengthen respiratory muscles.... boxers appreciate newfound ability to keep on punching....KB's reduce shoulder injuries....develop the ability to absorb ballistic shocks....build serious tendons and ligaments in wrists, elbows, shoulders, and back—with power to match....why kettlebell drills are better than plyometrics as a tool for developing power....KB's the tool of choice for rough sports.

Why Russian lifters train with kettlebells
Famous Soviet weightlifters start Olympic careers with KB's.... Olympic weightlifters add KB's for spectacular gains in shoulder and hip flexibility.... for developing quickness.... overhead kettlebell squats unmatchable in promoting hip and lower back flexibility for powerlifters.

Get huge with kettlebells—if you wish
Why the *girya* is superior to the dumbbell or barbell, for arm and chest training....how to gain muscle size doing KB C&J's.... repetition one arm snatches for bulking up your back, shoulders, and biceps.... Incorporating KB's into drop sets—for greater mass and vascularity.

Kettlebells for arm-wrestlers
World champion arm wrestler gives KB's two thumbs up....why the kettlebell is one of the best grip and forearm developers in existence....

Getting younger and healthier with kettlebells
The amazing health benefits of KB training.... Doctor Krayevskiy's 20-year age-reversal.... successful rehabilitation of hopeless back injuries with kettlebells.... Valentin Dikul—from broken back to All Time Historic Deadlift of 460kg, thanks to KB's....why KB's can be highly beneficial for your joints.

How kettlebells melt fat and build a powerful heart—without the dishonor of dieting and aerobics
Spectacular fat loss....enhanced metabolism.... increased growth hormone....a remarkable decrease in heart rates....

SECTION THREE
Doing It—Kettlebell Techniques and Programs for Xtreme Fitness

Why Kettlebells?
The many reasons to choose K-bells over mainstream equipment and methods.... KBs suitable for men and women young and old.... perfect for military, law enforcement and athletic teams....*Giryas*—a 'working class' answer to weightlifting and plyometrics promoting shoulder and hip flexibility....best bet for building best-at-show muscles....highly effective for strengthening the connective tissues....fixing bad backs....cheap and virtually indestructible....promotes genuine 'all-around fitness'—strength, explosiveness, flexibility, endurance, and fat loss.

The program minimum

The Russian Kettlebell Challenge workout: the program-maximum
Pavel's own free style program....the top ten Russian Kettlebell Challenge training guidelines....how often and how long to train.... The secret key to successful frequent training....THE most effective tool of strength development....difficulty and intensity variation....how to add *Power to the People!* and other drills to your kettlebell regimen

The kettlebell drills: *Explode!*
• **Swing/snatch pull**
• **Clean**—The key to efficient and painless shock absorption.... making the clean tougher....the pure evil of the two K-bells clean....seated hang cleans, for gorilla traps and shoulders....

• **Snatch**—The one-arm snatch—Tsar of kettlebell lifts
• **Under the leg pass**—A favorite of the Russian military—great for the midsection.
• **Jerk, Clean & Jerk**
• **Jump shrug**

The kettlebell drills: *Grind!*
• **Military press**—How to add and maximize tension for greater power....One hundred ways to cook the military press...The negative press....the 'powerlifter's secret weapon' for maximal results in your lifts....why to lift what you can't lift.... the graduated press.... how to get more out of a 'light' weight.... the two-kettlebells press....technique for building strength and muscle mass....the 'waiter press' for strict and perfect pressing skill....
• **Floor pullover and press**
• **Good morning stretch**—Favored by Russian weightlifters, for spectacular hamstring flexibility and hip strength.
• **Windmill**—An unreal drill for a powerful and flexible waist, back, and hips.
• **Side press**—A potent mix of the windmill and the military press—"one of the best builders of the shoulders and upper back."
• **Bent press**—A favorite lift of Eugene Sandow's—and The Evil One.... why the best-built men in history have been bent pressers....leads to proficiency in all other lifts....how to simultaneously use every muscle in your body.... A Brazilian Jiu Jitsu champion's personal kettlebell program

SECTION FOUR
Classic Kettlebell Programs from Mother Russia:

The official Soviet weightlifting textbook *girevoy sport* system of training

The *Weightlifting Yearbook girevoy sport* programs

Three official armed forces *girevoy sport* programs

Group training with kettlebells—Red Army style

Xtreme kettlebell training—Russian Navy SEAL style
Performing snatches and other explosive kettlebell drills under water....pseudo-isokinetic resistance.... how to make your muscle fibers blast into action faster than ever....

ANNOUNCING:

"The World's *Single Most Effective Tool* for Massive Gains in
Strength, Speed and Athletic Endurance"

- **Get thick, cable-like, hellaciously hard muscle**
- **Get frightening, whip-like speed**
- **Get stallion-like staying-power in any sport**
- **Get a, well, <u>god-like</u> physique**
- **Get the most brutal workout of your life, without having to leave your own living room**
- **Get way more energy in way less time**
- **Get a jack-rabbit's jumping power–and a jack-hammer's strength**
- **Get it all–and then more, with Russian KB's**

"Kettlebells are unsurpassed as a medium for increasing strength and explosive power. Thanks to Pavel Tsatsouline, I have now rewritten my training program to include kettlebell training, for athletes of all disciplines from Professional Football to Olympic sprinters."
—*Coach Davies*

*Discover why **Russian Kettlebells** are storming into "favored status" with US military, SWAT, NFL, MLB, powerlifters, weightlifters, martial artists–and elite athletes everywhere.*

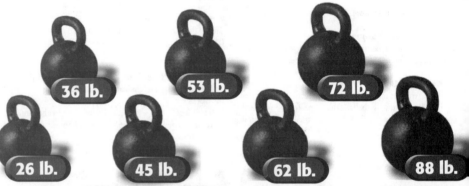

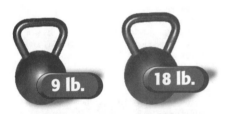

CLASSIC KETTLEBELLS

Each authentic Russian Kettlebell is manufactured exclusively by Dragon Door Publications in traditional weight sizes. The kettlebells are made out of solid cast iron and are coated in the highest quality scratch and rust resistant cathodic epoxy gloss. These kettlebells are designed to last a lifetime—and beyond.

Special warning: the *Russian Kettlebell* is an *Xtreme Edge Fitness* Tool for serious workout fiends. It is not a Barbie toy! Treat your kettlebell lifting with the utmost care, precision and respect. Watch Pavel's kettlebell video many, many times for perfect form and correct execution. If possible, sign up for one of Pavel's upcoming Kettlebell Training Bootcamp/Certification programs. Lift at your own discretion! We are not responsible for you boinking yourself on the head, dropping it on your feet or any other politically-incorrect action. Stick to the Party line, Comrade!

RUSSIAN KETTLEBELLS

STEEL HANDLE & CORE/RUBBER CASING	Price	MAIN USA	AK&HI	CAN
#P10D 4kg (approx. 9lb) —.25 poods	$89.95	S/H $10.00	$52.00	$29.00
#P10E 8kg (approx. 18lb) — .50 poods	$99.95	S/H $14.00	$70.00	$41.00

CLASSIC KETTLEBELLS (SOLID CAST IRON)

	Price	MAIN USA	AK&HI	CAN
#P10G 12kg (approx. 26lb) — .75 poods	$82.95	S/H $20.00	$86.00	$53.00
#P10A 16kg (approx. 36lb) — 1 pood	$89.95	S/H $24.00	$95.00	$65.00
#P10H 20kg (approx. 45lb) — 1.25 poods	$99.95	S/H $28.00	$118.00	$72.00
#P10B 24kg (approx. 53lb) — 1.5 poods	$109.95	S/H $32.00	$137.00	$89.00
#P10J 28kg (approx. 62lb) — 1.75 poods	$129.95	S/H $36.00	$154.00	$102.00
#P10C 32kg (approx. 72lb) — 2 poods	$139.95	S/H $39.00	$173.00	$115.00
#P10F 40kg (approx. 88lb) — 2.5 poods	$179.95	S/H $52.00	$210.00	$139.00

SAVE! ORDER A SET OF CLASSIC KETTLEBELLS & SAVE $17.00

		Price	MAIN USA	AK&HI	CAN
#SP10	Classic Set (one each of 16, 24 & 32kg)	$322.85	S/H $95.00	$405.00	$269.00

ALASKA/HAWAII KETTLEBELL ORDERING
Dragon Door now ships to all 50 states, including Alaska and Hawaii. We ship Kettlebells to Alaska and Hawaii via UPS 2nd Day Air service.

CANADIAN KETTLEBELL ORDERING
Dragon Door now accepts online, phone and mail orders for Kettlebells to Canada, using UPS Standard service. UPS Standard to Canada service is guaranteed, fully tracked ground delivery, available to every address in all of Canada's ten provinces. Delivery time can vary between 3 to 10 days.

<u>IMPORTANT</u> – International shipping quotes & orders do not include customs clearance, duties, taxes or other non-routine customs brokerage charges, which are the responsibility of the customer.

- **KETTLEBELLS ARE SHIPPED VIA UPS GROUND SERVICE, UNLESS OTHERWISE REQUESTED.**
- **KETTLEBELLS RANGING IN SIZE FROM 4KG TO 24KG CAN BE SHIPPED TO P.O. BOXES OR MILITARY ADDDRESSES VIA THE U.S. POSTAL SERVICE, BUT WE REQUIRE PHYSICAL ADDDRESSES FOR UPS DELIVERIES FOR THE 32KG AND 40KG KETTLEBELLS.**
- **<u>NO</u> RUSH ORDERS ON KETTLEBELLS!**

Russian Kettlebells—The Ultimate Iron Game for Massive, Massive, Massive, Massive, Massive
RESULTS

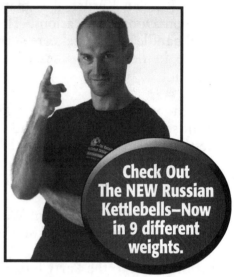

AMAZING NEWS:
Now You Can Carry a Whole Gym in One Hand—and Get a Fabulous,
TOTAL WORKOUT
Right in Your Own Living Room

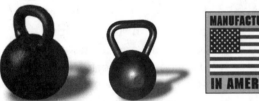

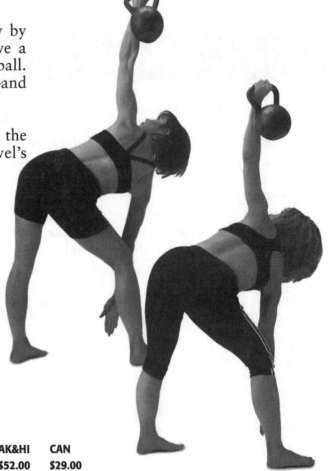

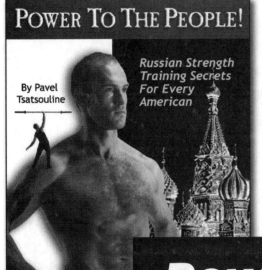

POWER TO THE PEOPLE!

RUSSIAN STRENGTH TRAINING SECRETS FOR EVERY AMERICAN

By Pavel Tsatsouline

8¹/₂" x 11" 124 pages, over 100 photographs and illustrations—$34.95 #B10

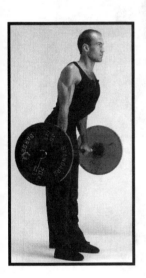

How would you like to own a world class body—<u>whatever your present condition</u>— by doing only two exercises, for twenty minutes a day?" A body so lean, ripped and powerful looking, you won't believe your own reflection when you catch yourself in the mirror.

And what if you could do it without a single supplement, without having to waste your time at a gym and with only a 150 bucks of simple equipment?

And how about not only being stronger than you've ever been in your life, but having higher energy and better performance in whatever you do?

How would you like to have an instant download of the world's <u>absolutely most effective strength secrets?</u> To possess exactly the same knowledge that created world-champion athletes—and the strongest bodies of their generation?"

Pavel Tsatsouline's *Power to the People!– Russian Strength Training Secrets for Every American* delivers all of this and more.

As Senior Science Editor for Joe Weider's *Flex* magazine, Jim Wright is recognized as one of the world's premier authorities on strength training. Here's more of what he had to say:
"*Whether you're young or old, a beginner or an elite athlete, training in your room or in the most high tech facility, if there was only one book I could recommend to help you reach your ultimate physical potential, this would be it.*

Simple, concise and truly reader friendly, this amazing book contains it all—everything you need to know—what exercises (only two!), how to do them (unique detailed information you'll find nowhere else), and why.

Follow its advice and, believe it or not, you'll be stronger and more injury-resistant immediately. I guarantee it. I only wish I'd had a book like this when I first began training.

Follow this program for three months and you'll not only be amazed but hooked. It is the ultimate program for "Everyman" AND Woman! I thought I knew a lot with a Ph.D. and 40 years of training experience...but I learned a lot and it's improved my training significantly."

And how about this from World Masters Powerlifting champion and Parrillo Performance Press editor, Marty Gallagher:

"*Pavel Tsatsouline has burst onto the American health and fitness scene like a Russian cyclone. He razes the sacred temples of fitness complacency and smugness with his revolutionary concepts and ideas. If you want a new and innovative approach to the age old dilemma of physical transformation, you've struck the mother-lode.*"

Here's just some of what you'll discover, when you possess your own copy of Pavel Tsatsouline's *Power to the People!*:

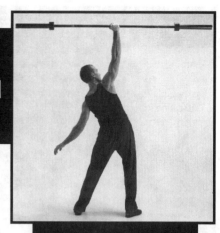

- How to get super strong without training to muscle failure or exhaustion
- How to hack into your 'muscle software' and magnify your power and muscle definition
- How to get super strong <u>without putting on an ounce of weight</u>
- Or how to build massive muscles with a classified Soviet Special Forces workout
- Why high rep training to the 'burn' is like a form of rigor mortis—and what it really takes to develop spectacular muscle tone
- How to mold your whole body into an off-planet rock with only two exercises
- How to increase your bench press by ten pounds overnight
- How to get a tremendous workout on the road without any equipment
- How to design a world class body in your basement—with $150 worth of basic weights and in twenty minutes a day
- How futuristic techniques can squeeze more horsepower out of your body-engine
- How to maximize muscular tension for traffic-stopping muscular definition
- How to minimize fatigue and get the most out of your strength training
- How to ensure high energy after your workout
- How to get stronger and harder without getting bigger
- Why it's safer to use free weights than machines
- How to achieve massive muscles <u>and</u> awesome strength—if that's what you want
- What, how and when to eat for maximum gains
- How to master the magic of effective exercise variation
- The ultimate formula for strength
- How to gain beyond your wildest dreams—with less chance of injury
- A high intensity, immediate gratification technique for massive strength gains
- The eight most effective breathing habits for lifting weights
- The secret that separates elite athletes from 'also-rans'
- How to become super strong and live to tell about it

"You are not training if you are not training with Pavel!"

—Dr. Fred Clary, National Powerlifting Champion and World Record Holder.

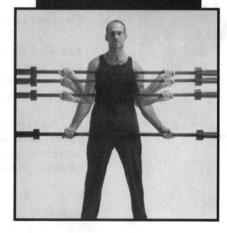

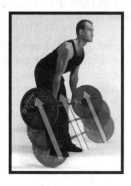

Russians have always made do with simple solutions without compromising the results. NASA aerospace types say that while America sends men to the moon in a Cadillac, Russia manages to launch them into space in a tin can. Enter the tin can approach to designing a world class body—in your basement with $150 worth of equipment. After all, US gyms are stuffed with hi-tech gear, yet it is the Russians with their metal junkyard training facilities who have dominated the Olympics for decades.

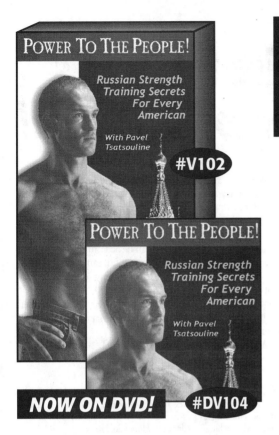

POWER TO THE PEOPLE

By Pavel Tsatsouline
Running time: 47 min

$29.95 Video #V102
$29.95 DVD #DV104

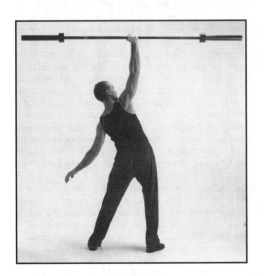

Now, It's Yours for the Taking: Irresistible Strength and a Body-to-Die-For

Turn on Pavel's Power to the People! video and watch in amazement as you rapidly increase your strength by 20, 30, even 50 percent—often in one session!

You may, or may not, want to startle your friends, excite your lovers, scare your enemies and paralyze your neighbors with envy, but believe me, it's gonna happen when you easily absorb Pavel's breakthrough strength secrets.

Of course, what's most important is how you're gonna feel about yourself. Get real! Toss out your lame rationalizations and pathetic excuses. Stop behaving like a spoilt brat about your infantile levels of strength. Stop hating yourself for banging your head against phony training plateaus. Now you can smash through the glass ceiling of your ignorance and burst into the higher reaches of maximum performance.

Let's face it—it's a delicious feeling to be as strong as a panther—confident, sure-of-yourself, genuinely attractive, a <u>SPECIMEN, THE GENUINE ARTICLE</u>, stalking the streets with evident power and natural grace.

I don't care who you are or what you are, I promise you: grab Pavel's Power to the People! video <u>IMMEDIATELY</u>, plug yourself in—and <u>I MEAN, PLUG YOURSELF IN</u>—do what it says, and you won't believe the new you.

Whatever your current workout program, just download Pavel's strength techniques for an immediate improvement in your results.

- Achieve super-strength without training to muscle failure or exhaustion
- Know the secret of hacking into your 'muscle software' to magnify power and muscle
- Get super strong without putting on an ounce of weight
- Discover what it really takes to develop spectacular muscle tone
- Discover how to mold your whole body into an off-planet rock with only two exercises
- Now you can design a world class body in your basement—with $150 worth of basic weights and in twenty minutes a day
- Discover futuristic techniques to squeeze more horsepower out of your body-engine
- Discover how to maximize muscular tension and get traffic-stopping muscular definition
- Learn why it's safer to use free weights than machines
- How to achieve massive muscles and awesome strength—if that's what you want
- How to master the magic of effective exercise variation
- Know how to gain beyond your wildest dreams—with less chance of injury
- Discover a high intensity, immediate gratification technique for massive strength gains
- Discover the eight most effective breathing habits for lifting weights
- Learn the secret that separates elite athletes from 'also-rans'

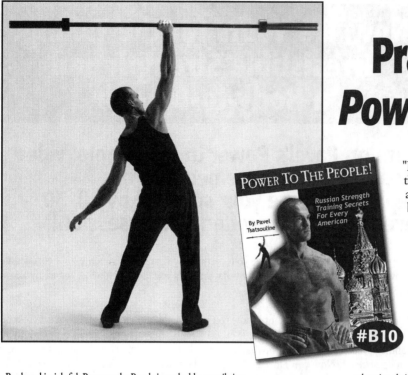

Praise for Pavel's Power to the People!

"In **Power to the People!** Pavel Tsatsouline reveals an authentically Russian approach to physical fitness. He shows how anyone, by learning how to contract their muscles harder, can build up to incredible levels of strength without gaining an ounce of weight. He shows how to exercise with a super-strict form and lift more weight than can be accomplished by swing or cheat. Now it's possible to train the human body to world-class fitness standards at home, working out for twenty minutes a day, and with only $150.00 worth of basic weights. **Power to the People!** is a highly recommended addition to any personal or professional physical fitness reference bookshelf."
—Midwest Book Review, Oregon, WI

Brash and insightful, Power to the People is a valuable compilation of how-to strength training information. Pavel Tsatsouline offers a fresh and provocative perspective on resistance training, and charts a path to self-improvement that is both practical and elegantly simple. If building strength is your top priority, then *Power to the People* belongs at the top of your reading list. —Rob Faigin, author of Natural Hormonal Enhancement

"I learned a lot from Pavel's books and plan to use many of his ideas in my own workouts. *Power to the People!* is an eye-opener. It will give you new—and valuable—perspectives on strength training. You will find plenty of ideas here to make your training more productive."—Clarence Bass, author of Ripped 1, 2 &3.

"A good book for the athlete looking for a routine that will increase strength without building muscle mass. Good source of variation for anyone who's tired of doing standard exercises."—Jonathan Lawson, IronMan Magazine

"I have been a training athlete for over 30 years. I played NCAA basketball in college, kick boxed as a pro for two years, made it to the NFL as a free agent in 1982, powerlifted through my 20's and do Olympic lifting now at 42. I have also coached swimming and strength athletes for over 20 years.I have never read a book more useful than **Power to the People!** I have seen my strength explode like I was in my 20's again—and my joints are no longer hurting."—Carter Stamm, New Orleans, LA

"I have been following a regimen I got from *Power to the People!* for about seven weeks now. I have lost about 17lbs and have lost three inches in my waist. My deadlift has gone from a meager 180lbs to 255 lbs in that short time as well."—Lawrence J. Kochert

"Like *Beyond Stretching* and *Beyond Crunches*, his other books, this is great. I think that it is the best book on effective strength training that I have ever read. This is not a book just about theory and principles. But Tsatsouline provides a detailed and complete outline of an exact program to do and how to customize it for yourself. It is very different from anything you have probably every read about strength training. The things he teaches in the book though won't just get you strong, if you want more than that, but can make you look really good—lean, ripped, and/or real big muscled if you want it. It's a very good book; the best available English-language print matter on the topic of strength training."—Dan Paltzik

"The great thing about the book *"Power to the People!"* is that it tells the readers what not to do when training for strength and why not. As you read the book, you will keep saying to yourself: "so that's why I'm not getting stronger!" Pavel points out all the things that are wrong with conventional weight training (and there is lots of it) and shows the readers what they need to do to get stronger, but not necessarily bigger."— Sang Kim, Rome, GA

"Using Pavel Tsatsouline's weight training methods from his book *Power to the People* gives you the feeling that you can take on the world after only a 20-30 minute workout! Tsatsouline's book is written with such cleverness, clarity, and detail that I couldn't put it down. I am thoroughly enthusiastic about weight training where my past indoor training consisted only of Yoga postures. I would recommend this book to anyone interested in enhancing their performance on the job, in weight training, and in other athletic pursuits. Pavel's genius is that he can take a complex subject like weight training and design a program that is enjoyable, efficient and gets fast results. He has done the same thing for abdominal development and stretching."—Cliff D.V., Honolulu, Hawaii

"I have experienced Pavel Tsatsouline's methods up close and in person, and his scientific approach lays waste to the muscleheaded garbage that we've been conditioned to follow. Pavel will show you how to achieve a full-body workout with just two core exercises and $150 worth of barbell equipment. You won't get injured and you won't get stiff. You'll just get what you were looking for in the first place - a program that works and one that you'll stick with." — David M Gaynes, Bellevue, WA

"It isn't growth hormone... it's Pavel! This is THE definitive text on the art and science of strength training... and that's what it's all about, power! Page after page of the world's most useful and productive strength-training practices are explained in this book. A lot of experienced lifters, who think that they know how to train, will be humbled when they find out how much better Pavel's system is than anything the western iron-game community has ever done. I have surpassed all my previous bests...and I no longer need or use lifting belts. I learned how to up-regulate tension through his "feed-forward" technique, how to immediately add AT LEAST ten pounds to every lift via "hyperirradiation", and to do it in my best form ever, and how to gain on every lift WEEKLY through the Russian system of periodization without any plateaus! Seriously, I gain every week! You only need TWO exercises! Pavel explains which ones, how to do them and how often. Also, you'll learn how to train to SUCCESS, not to "failure", how to immediately turn any lift into a "hyper lift", teach your nervous system how not to ever "miss" a lift, and simultaneously make your body far less injury-prone! Pavel illustrates the two types of muscle growth and which one you REALLY need, and the all-important power breathing. Pavel's training is the most valuable resource made available for strength athletes since the barbell. The breathing techniques alone are worth the asking price. This book is my personal favorite out of all his works, and in my opinion, they should be owned as a set. This book is superior to all the muscle mags and books that dwell on a content of unessential details of today's "fitness culture" and yet never fully explain the context of training for strength. Pavel cuts right to the heart of the "muscle mystery", by explaining the all-important context of the Russian system: quick, efficient, permanent strength gains, without spending a small fortune on "me-too" bodybuilding supplements and without unnecessary, time consuming overtraining. Now I only hope he writes a book on full-contact training..."—Sean Williams, Long Beach, NY

"This is a real source of no-b.s. information on how to build strength without adding bulk. I learned some new things which one can't find in books like *'Beyond Brawn'* or *'Dinosaur Training'*. Perhaps an advanced powerlifter, who reads Milo, already knows all that stuff, but I would definitely recommend this book to everyone from beginners to intermediates who are interested in increasing their strength." —Nikolai Pastouchenko, Tallahassee, Florid

"Forget all of the fancy rhetoric. If you are serious about improving your strength and your health buy this book and pay attention to what's provided. I started in January 2000 doing deadlifts with 200 lbs. Three months later I was at 365 lbs. Pavel knows what he is talking about and knows how to explain it simply. That's it."—Alan, Indiana

The Graduate Course In Instant Strength Gains

"I went from 5 to 10 pullups in one week."

"Last night I did 15 one-arm pushups with each arm. Two months ago I couldn't do one complete rep."

"I could do one wobbly one-legged squat… [Two weeks later] I did 5 clean, butt-to-ground pistols."

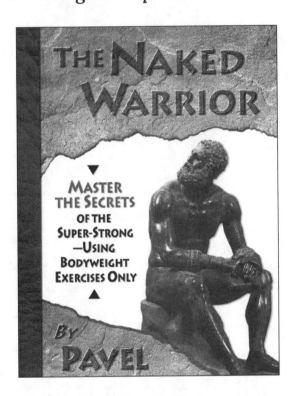

The Naked Warrior
Master the Secrets of the Super-Strong—Using Bodyweight Exercises Only
By Pavel Tsatsouline

#B28 $39.95
Paperback   218 pages   8.5" x 11"
Over 190 black & white photos
plus several illustrations

Have you noticed—the greater a man's skill, the more he achieves with less? And the skill of strength is no exception. From the ancient days of Greek wrestling, to the jealously guarded secrets of Chinese Kung Fu masters, to the hard men of modern spec ops, warriors and allied strongmen have developed an amazing array of skills for generating inhuman strength.

But these skills have been scattered far and wide, held closely secret, or communicated in a piecemeal fashion that has left most of us frustrated and far from reaching our true strength potential.

Now, for the first time, Russian strength expert and former *Spetsnaz* instructor Pavel has gathered many of these devastating techniques into one highly teachable skill set. In *The Naked Warrior* Pavel reveals exactly what it takes to be super-strong in minimum time—when your body is your only tool.

Praise for Pavel's *The Naked Warrior*

"As a diehard weightlifting competitor throughout the past 40 years, I at first viewed the bodyweight-only approach of *The Naked Warrior* with some trepidation. Imagine my surprise when discovering Pavel Tsatsouline's latest work stresses real STRENGTH TRAINING, employment of a limited amount of key major muscle group movements, and a high intensity, low rep format! Indeed, by deriving the best features of proven power building programs from all weightlifting disciplines, gymnastics, martial arts, and other "heavy" exercise modes, Mr. Tsatsouline has redefined strength-conditioning for the 21st century!

Recently retired from 32 years in public education, I used to agonize over the archaic athletic training which was witnessed on a daily basis; coaches simply led their charges through hours of mind-numbing, ineffective calisthenics, "tradition" since centuries before. Now, Pavel's research can yield a much more condensed, result- producing package. *The Naked Warrior* routine has the potential to save teams huge blocks of much needed time, will not drain their athletes' energy, and saves from any strain on the usual tight budget—no new equipment, definitely no assembly required!!!"
—**John McKean, six time All-Round Weightlifting World Champion**

"Pavel... your sections on tension and breathing de-mystify the concept of 'centering'. Many practitioners of Oriental arts emphasize the mental path to power generation. The majority of Westerners cannot relate to that. You have made it a physical skill and described it in such a way that anyone can practice it and readily improve... This book, as with *The Russian Kettlebell Challenge...* will catch like fire in the tactical community."
—**Name withheld, Instructor, Counter Assault Team, US Secret Service**

"If I was stuck on a desert island (or somewhere else with no access to weights) I'd hope that Pavel Tsatsouline would be there to help keep me in shape. With *The Naked Warrior*, Pavel has moved the art of exercise without weights to a new level. I like both the exercises he has selected and the approach he advocates for training on them. Now, whether you have weights or not, there is no reason not to get into top shape!"
—**Arthur Drechsler, author "The Weightlifting Encyclopedia"**

The Naked Warrior
Master the Secrets of the Super-Strong—Using Bodyweight Exercises Only
By Pavel Tsatsouline

#B28 $39.95
Paperback   218 pages   8.5" x 11"
Over 190 black & white photos

"This book has caused me to completely re-evaluate the way I look at calisthenics... Education is a wonderful thing and in this book you have most certainly educated me, as you will educate thousands... The great detail you include works, as I often receive a great deal of e-mail asking for more detail. Even those of us who have cranked out hundreds of thousands of reps in various drills don't really know what we are doing at a micro level. The detail allows us to scrutinize our performance and make adjustments to improve performance.

As for the spec ops warrior, this is great! There are so many times when you are unable to bring weights with you and you have to rely on cals to get you through.

This new learning on cals allows us in the field to still train for great strength with only our bodies and that's like money in the bank! For example, I am going on a 10 day trip with no weights and I will most certainly do *The Naked Warrior* workout while I am gone! I can't wait to get started!

The Naked Warrior is a must for anyone who trains people with cals! While it's great for your own use, you can help others improve dramatically by knowing what to look for and what to suggest to improve their technique."
—**SSgt. Nate Morrison, USAF, Pararescue Combatives Course Project Manager**

"*The Naked Warrior* is one of Pavel's best work yet!!! I find that Pavel's easy to understand, no nonsense approach in *The Naked Warrior* will help one become the best they can be. In addition, the tools Pavel explains in *The Naked Warrior* will help my Olympic style weight lifters gain the core strength they need to put additional kg on their totals. Thanks Pavel for such a great work!!"
—**Mike Burgener, Sr international weightlifting coach**

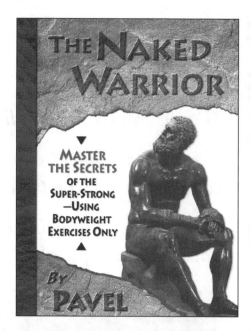

"*The Naked Warrior* is outstanding as a complement to Pavel's other books or standing alone. The 'Grease the Groove' section alone makes this book worth owning. For martial artists and practitioners of police defensive tactics the two featured exercises in *The Naked Warrior* will greatly enhance striking and kicking. The One-Arm Pushup and the One-Legged Squat (Pistol) are the closest thing to actually striking and kicking that strength training has to offer.

For martial artists who don't wish to weight train or just don't have the time *The Naked Warrior* program is the way to go to enhance strength. Those who do weight train will want to include the Naked Warrior program into their training as well since the benefit is great while time, cost and convenience are non-factors.

The 'byproduct' of the high tension concepts outlined in this book is the martial artist will learn more about the use of muscle tension in motion than he will during the majority of martial arts training. Tension, in it's proper degree and application is of paramount importance, it is not only a factor in strength, but in speed and endurance as well. The section on Power Breathing explains the relation between strength and breathing like most martial art instructors don't or cannot.

There is finally a scientific explanation on many of the breathing exercises and techniques that abound. As is stated in the book, 'strength is a technique.' You can practice martial skills without the information offered in *The Naked Warrior*, but you risk not operating at full potential."
—**George Demetriou, Modern Warrior**

Highlights Of What You Get With Pavel's *The Naked Warrior*

Chapter 1
The Naked Warrior Rules of Engagement

'The Naked Warrior', or why strength train with bodyweight? The definition of strength...strength classifications...examples of the three types of strength...the only way to build strength...high resistance and mental focus on contraction ...tension generation skill...a powerful instant-strength mix...The Naked Warrior Principles ...the six keys to greater strength...How do lifters really train?...'best practice' secrets of powerlifters and Olympic weightlifters...How do gymnasts get a good workout with the same weight?...five strategies for making 5-rep exercises harder...how gymnasts achieve super strength...how to customize the resistance without changing the weight.

Chapter 2
The Naked Warrior Workout

"Grease the groove," or how to get superstrong without a routine...the secret success formula...Some GTG testimonials from the dragondoor.com forum...how does the GTG system work?...turning your nerves into superconductors...avoiding muscle failure... strength as a skill—the magic formula..."The Pistol": the Russian Spec Ops' leg strengthener of choice...how to do it—the basics...The one-arm/one-leg pushup: "an exercise in total body tension"...what gymnastics has to teach us...another advantage of the one-arm pushup...GTG, the ultimate specialization program.

Chapter 3
High-Tension Techniques for Instant Strength

Tension. What force is made of...the relationship between tension and force...high-tension techniques...'Raw strength' versus 'technique' ...the power of mental focus...Low gear for brute force...speed and tension...putting explosiveness in context..."Doesn't dynamic tension act like a brake?"... a dirty little secret of bodybuilding ...the dangers of mindless lifting...The power of a fist...the principle of irradiation...Accidental discharge of strength: a tip from firearms instructors...interlimb response and your muscle software...Power abs = a power body...the relationship between abs tension and body strength... he 'back-pressure crunch'...the source of real striking power...A gymnast instantly gains 40 pounds of strength on his iron cross with the three techniques you have just learned...The "static stomp": using ground pressure to maximize power...a secret of top karatekas and bench pressers...how the secret of armpit power translates into paydirt for one-arm pushups, punches, and bench presses..."The corkscrew":

Another secret of the karate punch...the power of rotation and spiral...the invisible force...Bracing: boost your strength up to 20% with an armwrestling tactic...when to brace...the advantage of dead-start exercises...'Body hardening'—tough love for teaching tension...the quick and hard way to greater tension control...Beyond bracing: "zipping up"...taking your pretensing skills to a new level...Wind up for power...the art of storing elastic energy for greater power...the reverse squat.

Chapter 4
Power Breathing: The Martial Arts Masters' Secret for Superstrength

Bruce Lee called it "breath strength"...cranking up your breath strength...your body as a first-class sound system—how to make it happen... definition of true power breathing...Power inhalation...the mystery breathing muscle that's vital to your strength...amping up the compression...when and why to hold your breath...Reverse power breathing: evolution of the Iron Shirt technique...the pelvic diaphragm lock...two crucial rules for maximal power breathing...Power up from the core, or the 'pneumatics of Chi'...two important principles of power generation...how to avoid a power leakage...the "balloon" technique for greater power.

Chapter 5
Driving GTG Home

Driving GTG home: focused...skill-building— why "fewer is better"...the law of the jungle...Driving GTG home: flawless...how to achieve perfection—the real key...the five conditions for generating high tension...the significance of low rep work...Driving GTG home: frequent...the one great secret of press success...Driving GTG home: fresh...the many aspects of staying fresh for optimal strength gains...staying away from failure...the balancing act between frequency and freshness...Driving GTG home: fluctuating...how to avoid training plateaus..."same yet different" strategies... 'waviness of load'...countering fatigue...training guidelines for a PR...backing off and overtraining.

Chapter 6
Field-Stripping the Pistol

Box Pistol...how to go from zero to hero...the box squat—a champions' favorite for multi-muscle strength gains...making a quantum leap in your squats...various options from easier to eviler...the rocking pistol...how to recruit your hip flexors...how to avoid cramping...One-Legged Squat, Paul Anderson style...Airborne Lunge...Pistol Classic...mastering the real

deal...Negative-Free Pistol...the three advantages of concentric-only training...Renegade Pistol ...Fire-in-the-Hole Pistol ... Cossack Pistol ...Dynamic Isometric Pistol...combining dynamic exercise with high-tension stops...multiple stops for greater pain...taking advantage of your sticking points...easier variations...three reasons why adding isos to dynamic lifting can increase effectiveness by up to 15%...protecting yourself against injury...Isometric Pistol...holding tension over time...the art of "powered-down" high-tension techniques...Weighted Pistol...working the spinal erectors.

Chapter 7
Field-Stripping the One-Arm Pushup

The One-Arm Pushup, floor and elevated...how to shine at high-intensity exertion...change-ups for easy and difficult...the authorized technique...developing a controlled descent... Isometric One-Arm Pushup...The One-Arm Dive Bomber Pushup...The One-Arm Pump...The One-Arm Half Bomber Pushup...Four more drills to work up to the One-Arm Dive Bomber...The One-Arm/One-Leg Pushup...the Tsar of the one-arm pushups.

Chapter 8
Naked Warrior Q&A

Are bodyweight exercises superior to exercises with weights?...the advantage of cals...what cals enforce...the biggest disadvantage of bodyweight exercising...the advantage of barbells...the advantages and disadvantages of dumbbells...the advantages of kettlebells...Why is there such an intense argument in the martial arts community as to whether bodyweight exercises are superior to exercises with weights?...confusions explained ...what a fighter needs...Can I get very strong using only bodyweight exercises?...Should I mix different strength-training tools in my training? ...How can I incorporate bodyweight exercises with kettlebell and barbell training?...Can the high-tension techniques and GTG system be applied to weights?... Can the high-tension techniques and GTG system be applied to strength endurance training?...I can't help overtraining. What should I do?...Can I follow the Naked Warrior program on an ongoing basis?...Can I add more exercises to the Naked Warrior program?...Will my development be unbalanced from doing only two exercises?...Is there a way to work the lats with a pulling exercise when no weights or pullup bars are accessible?...door pullups...door rows...Where can I learn more about bodyweight-only strength training?...Low reps and no failure? This training is too easy!...Will I forget all the strength techniques in some sort of emergency?...Isn't dedicating most of the book to technique too much?...why technique is crucial...moving from ordinary to extraordinary.

Get RAW, Get POTENT, Get POWERFUL—

When You Unleash the Power of Instinctual Eating

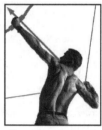

Eat like an emperor—and have a gladiator's body

Are you still confused about what, how and when to eat? Despite the diet books you have read and the programs you have tried, do you still find yourself lacking in energy, carrying excess body fat, and feeling physically run-down? Sexually, do you feel a shadow of your former self?

The problem, according to **Ori Hofmekler**, is that we have lost touch with the natural wisdom of our instinctual drives. We have become the slaves of our own creature comforts—scavenger/victims rather than predator/victors. When to comes to informed-choice, we lack any real sense of personal freedom. The result: ill-advised eating and lifestyle habits that leave us vulnerable to all manner of disease—not to mention obesity and sub-par performance.

The Warrior Diet presents a brilliant and far-reaching solution to our nutritional woes, based on a return to the primal power of our natural instincts.

The first step is to break the chains of our current eating habits. Drawing on a combination of ancient history and modern science, *The Warrior Diet* proves that humans are at their energetic, physical, mental and passionate best when they "undereat" during the day and "overeat" at night. Once you master this essential eating cycle, a new life of explosive vigor and vitality will be yours for the taking.

Unlike so many dietary gurus, Ori Hofmekler has personally followed his diet for over twenty-five years and is a perfect model of *the Warrior Diet's* success—the man is a human dynamo.

Not just a diet, but a whole way of life, *the Warrior Diet* encourages us to seize back the pleasures of being alive—from the most refined to the wild and raw. *The Warrior Diet* is practical, tested, and based in commonsense. Expect results!

The Warrior Diet covers all the bases. As an added bonus, discover delicious Warrior Recipes, a special Warrior Workout, and a line of Warrior Supplements—designed to give you every advantage in the transformation of your life from average to exceptional.

The Warrior Diet
Switch On Your Biological Powerhouse—For Explosive Strength, High Energy and a Leaner, Harder Body
By Ori Hofmekler With Diana Holtzberg

#B23 $24.00
Paperback 420 pages 6" x 9"
#B17 $26.95
Hardcover 420 pages 5 3/8" x 8 3/8"
Over 150 photographs and illustrations

About Ori Hofmekler

Ori Hofmekler is a modern Renaissance man whose life has been driven by two passions: art and sports. Hofmekler's formative experience as a young man with the Israeli Special Forces, prompted a lifetime's interest in diets and fitness regimes that would optimize his physical and mental performance.

After the army, Ori attended the Bezalel Academy of Art and the Hebrew University, where he studied art and philosophy and received a degree in Human Sciences.

A world-renowned painter, best known for his controversial political satire, Ori's work has been featured in magazines worldwide, including *Time, Newsweek, Rolling Stone, People, The New Republic* as well as *Penthouse* where he was a monthly columnist for 17 years and Health Editor from 1998–2000. Ori has published two books of political art, *Hofmekler's People*, and *Hofmekler's Gallery*.

As founder, Editor-In-Chief, and Publisher of *Mind & Muscle Power*, a national men's health and fitness magazine, Ori introduced his Warrior Diet to the public in a monthly column—to immediate acclaim from readers and professionals in the health industry alike.

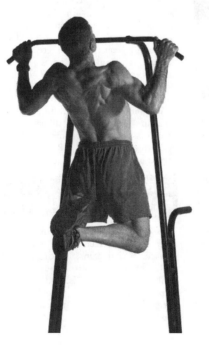

Acclaim for The Warrior Diet

"For those individuals who like to think outside of the box, *The Warrior Diet* represents an innovative approach to fitness and weight loss. No questions, it's worked for Ori Hofmekler, so why not give it a shot?"

—Men's Exercise, Aug 2003

"In a startling reversal of recent dietary advice fitness expert Ori shows how you can indeed have your cake and eat it too—staying slim and trim while indulging yourself with many of your favorite foods. Not just another diet book, *The Warrior Diet* presents a brilliant synthesis of modern scientific research and ancient time-tested secrets for reducing body fat, gaining energy and looking younger."

—Women's Health and Fitness, June 2003

"In my quest for a lean, muscular body, I have seen practically every diet and suffered through most of them. It is also my business to help others with their fat loss programs. I am supremely skeptical of any eating plan or "diet" book that can't tell me how and why it works in simple language. Ori Hofmekler's *The Warrior Diet* does just this, with a logical, readable approach that provides grounding for his claims and never asks the reader to take a leap of faith. *The Warrior Diet* can be a very valuable weapon in the personal arsenal of any woman."

—DC Maxwell, 2-time Women's Brazilian Jiu-Jitsu World Champion, Co-Owner, Maxercise Sports/Fitness Training Center and Relson Gracie Jiu-Jitsu Academy East

"The information in *The Warrior Diet* will help you achieve the next level in training for the 21st century. It is the physical training along with the diet that will make a lasting impact on your life. I am deeply grateful for Ori's advice and the friendship we have established over the years."

—Sifu John R. Salgado, World Champion, Chinese Wrestling and Taiji Push Hands

"*The Warrior Diet* certainly defies so-called modern nutritional and training dogmas.

Having met Ori on several occasions, I can certainly attest that he is the living proof that his system works. He maintains a ripped muscular body year round despite juggling extreme workloads and family life. His take on supplementation is refreshing as he promotes an integrated and timed approach. *The Warrior Diet* is a must read for the nutrition and training enthusiast who wishes to expand his horizons."

—Charles Poliquin, author of *The Poliquin Principles* and *Modern Trends in Strength Training*, Three-Time Olympic Strength Coach

"Despite its name, *The Warrior Diet* isn't about leading a Spartan lifestyle, although it is about improving quality of life. With a uniquely compelling approach, the book guides you towards the body you want by re-awakening primal instinct and biofeedback—the things that have allowed us to evolve this far. Ironically, in a comfortable world of overindulgence, your survival may still be determined by natural selection. If this is the case, *The Warrior Diet* will be the only tool you'll need."

—Brian Batcheldor, Science writer/researcher, National Coach, British Powerlifting Team

"In a era of decadence, where wants and desires are virtually limitless, Ori's vision recalls an age of warriors, where success meant survival and survival was the only option. A diet of the utmost challenge from which users will reap tremendous benefits."

—John Davies, Olympic and professional sports strength/speed coach

"Ori Hofmekler has his finger on a deep, ancient and very visceral pulse—one that too many of us have all but forgotten. Part warrior-athlete, part philosopher-romantic, Ori not only reminds us what this innate, instinctive rhythm is all about, he also shows us how to detect and rekindle it in our own bodies. His program challenges and guides each of us to fully reclaim for ourselves the

strength, sinew, energy and spirit that humans have always been meant to possess."

—Pilar Gerasimo, Editor in Chief, *Experience Life Magazine*

"I refuse to graze all day, I have better things to do. I choose *The Warrior Diet*."

—Pavel Tsatsouline, author of *Power to the People!* and *The Russian Kettlebell Challenge*

"I think of myself as a modern-day warrior; businessman, family man and competitive athlete. In the 2 years that I have been following *The Warrior Diet*, I have enjoyed the predators' advantage of freedom from the necessity of frequent feedings. I also benefit from the competitive edge of being a fat burning machine. My 12-year-old son, who is also a competitive athlete, has naturally gravitated towards *The Warrior Diet*. He is growing up lean, strong and healthy, unlike many of his peers, many of whom, even in this land of plenty, are overweight and frequently sick. Thank you, Ori, for writing *The Warrior Diet*."

—Stephen Maxwell, Ms., 2-time Brazilian Jiu-Jitsu World Champion, Co-Owner, Maxercise Sports/Fitness Training Center and Relson Gracie Jiu-Jitsu Academy East

"My body continues to get tighter and more toned in all of the right places...and people marvel at my eating practices.

Read *The Warrior Diet* with an open mind. Digest the information at your own pace. Assimilate the knowledge to make it fit into your current lifestyle. You will be amazed at how much more productive and energetic you will be. Be a warrior in your own right. Your body will thank you for it."

—Laura Moore, Science writer, *Penthouse* Magazine, *IronMan* Magazine, Body of the Month for IronMan, Sept 2001, Radio Talk Show Host *The Health Nuts*, author of *Sex Heals*

ORDERING INFORMATION

Customer Service Questions? Please call us between 9:00am–11:00pm EST Monday to Friday at 1-800-899-5111. Local and foreign customers call 513-346-4160 for orders and customer service

100% One-Year Risk-Free Guarantee. If you are not completely satisfied with any product–for any reason, no matter how long after you received it–we'll be happy to give you a prompt exchange, credit, or refund, as you wish. Simply return your purchase to us, and please let us know why you were dissatisfied–it will help us to provide better products and services in the future. *Shipping and handling fees are non-refundable.*

Telephone Orders For faster service you may place your orders by calling Toll Free 24 hours a day, 7 days a week, 365 days per year. When you call, please have your credit card ready.

1·800·899·5111
24 HOURS A DAY
FAX YOUR ORDER (866) 280-7619

Complete and mail with full payment to: Dragon Door Publications, P.O. Box 1097, West Chester, OH 45071

Please print clearly

Sold To: **A**

Name_____

Street_____

City_____

State _____ Zip _____

Day phone*_____
* Important for clarifying questions on orders

Please print clearly

SHIP TO: *(Street address for delivery)*   **B**

Name_____

Street_____

City_____

State _____ Zip _____

Email_____

ITEM #	QTY.	ITEM DESCRIPTION	ITEM PRICE	A OR B	TOTAL

HANDLING AND SHIPPING CHARGES · NO COD'S
Total Amount of Order Add:

$00.00 to $24.99 add $5.00	$100.00 to $129.99 add $12.00
$25.00 to $39.99 add $6.00	$130.00 to $169.99 add $14.00
$40.00 to $59.99 add $7.00	$170.00 to $199.99 add $16.00
$60.00 to $99.99	$200.00 to $299.99 add $18.00
	$300.00 and up add $20.00

Canada & Mexico add $8.00. All other countries triple U.S. charges.

Total of Goods	
Shipping Charges	
Rush Charges	
Kettlebell Shipping Charges	
OH residents add 6% sales tax	
MN residents add 6.5% sales tax	
TOTAL ENCLOSED	

METHOD OF PAYMENT ❑ CHECK ❑ M.O. ❑ MASTERCARD ❑ VISA ❑ DISCOVER ❑ AMEX

Account No. *(Please indicate all the numbers on your credit card)*   EXPIRATION DATE

☐☐☐☐ ☐☐☐☐ ☐☐☐☐ ☐☐☐☐   ☐☐/☐☐

Day Phone ( ) _____

SIGNATURE _____   DATE _____

NOTE: We ship best method available for your delivery address. Foreign orders are sent by air. Credit card or International M.O. only. For rush processing of your order, add an additional $10.00 per address. Available on money order & charge card orders only.

Errors and omissions excepted. Prices subject to change without notice.

ORDERING INFORMATION

Customer Service Questions? Please call us between 9:00am–11:00pm EST Monday to Friday at 1-800-899-5111. Local and foreign customers call 513-346-4160 for orders and customer service

100% One-Year Risk-Free Guarantee. If you are not completely satisfied with any product–for any reason, no matter how long after you received it–we'll be happy to give you a prompt exchange, credit, or refund, as you wish. Simply return your purchase to us, and please let us know why you were dissatisfied–it will help us to provide better products and services in the future. *Shipping and handling fees are non-refundable.*

Telephone Orders For faster service you may place your orders by calling Toll Free 24 hours a day, 7 days a week, 365 days per year. When you call, please have your credit card ready.

1·800·899·5111
24 HOURS A DAY
FAX YOUR ORDER (866) 280-7619

Complete and mail with full payment to: Dragon Door Publications, P.O. Box 1097, West Chester, OH 45071

Please print clearly

Sold To: **A**

Name_____

Street_____

City_____

State _____ Zip _____

Day phone*_____
Important for clarifying questions on orders

Please print clearly

SHIP TO: *(Street address for delivery)* **B**

Name_____

Street_____

City_____

State _____ Zip _____

Email_____

Warning to foreign customers:
The Customs in your country may or may not tax or otherwise charge you an additional fee for goods you receive. Dragon Door Publications is charging you only for U.S. handling and international shipping. Dragon Door Publications is in no way responsible for any additional fees levied by Customs, the carrier or any other entity.

ITEM #	QTY.	ITEM DESCRIPTION	ITEM PRICE	A OR B	TOTAL

HANDLING AND SHIPPING CHARGES • NO COD'S
Total Amount of Order Add:

$00.00 to $24.99 add $5.00	$100.00 to $129.99 add $12.00
$25.00 to $39.99 add $6.00	$130.00 to $169.99 add $14.00
$40.00 to $59.99 add $7.00	$170.00 to $199.99 add $16.00
$60.00 to $99.99 add $10.00	$200.00 to $299.99 add $18.00
	$300.00 and up add $20.00

Canada & Mexico add $8.00. All other countries triple U.S. charges.

Total of Goods	
Shipping Charges	
Rush Charges	
Kettlebell Shipping Charges	
OH residents add 6% sales tax	
MN residents add 6.5% sales tax	
TOTAL ENCLOSED	

METHOD OF PAYMENT ❏ CHECK ❏ M.O. ❏ MASTERCARD ❏ VISA ❏ DISCOVER ❏ AMEX

Account No. *(Please indicate all the numbers on your credit card)*   EXPIRATION DATE

❏❏❏❏ ❏❏❏❏ ❏❏❏❏ ❏❏❏❏   ❏❏/❏❏

Day Phone (   )_____

SIGNATURE _____ DATE _____

NOTE: We ship best method available for your delivery address. Foreign orders are sent by air. Credit card or International M.O. only. For rush processing of your order, add an additional $10.00 per address. Available on money order & charge card orders only.

Errors and omissions excepted. Prices subject to change without notice.

DDP 03/04

ORDERING INFORMATION

Customer Service Questions? Please call us between 9:00am–11:00pm EST Monday to Friday at 1-800-899-5111. Local and foreign customers call 513-346-4160 for orders and customer service

100% One-Year Risk-Free Guarantee. If you are not completely satisfied with any product–for any reason, no matter how long after you received it–we'll be happy to give you a prompt exchange, credit, or refund, as you wish. Simply return your purchase to us, and please let us know why you were dissatisfied–it will help us to provide better products and services in the future. *Shipping and handling fees are non-refundable.*

Telephone Orders For faster service you may place your orders by calling Toll Free 24 hours a day, 7 days a week, 365 days per year. When you call, please have your credit card ready.

1•800•899•5111
24 HOURS A DAY
FAX YOUR ORDER (866) 280-7619

Complete and mail with full payment to: Dragon Door Publications, P.O. Box 1097, West Chester, OH 45071

Please print clearly
Sold To: A

Name_____

Street_____

City_____

State _____ Zip _____

Day phone*_____
* Important for clarifying questions on orders

Please print clearly
SHIP TO: *(Street address for delivery)*   B

Name_____

Street_____

City_____

State _____ Zip _____

Email _____

Item #	Qty.	Item Description	Item Price	A or B	Total

HANDLING AND SHIPPING CHARGES • NO COD'S
Total Amount of Order Add:

$00.00 to $24.99 add $5.00	$100.00 to $129.99 add $12.00
$25.00 to $39.99 add $6.00	$130.00 to $169.99 add $14.00
$40.00 to $59.99 add $7.00	$170.00 to $199.99 add $16.00
$60.00 to $99.99	$200.00 to $299.99 add $18.00
	$300.00 and up add $20.00

Canada & Mexico add $8.00. All other countries triple U.S. charges.

Total of Goods	
Shipping Charges	
Rush Charges	
Kettlebell Shipping Charges	
OH residents add 6% sales tax	
MN residents add 6.5% sales tax	
Total Enclosed	

Method of Payment ❏ Check ❏ M.O. ❏ Mastercard ❏ Visa ❏ Discover ❏ Amex

Account No. *(Please indicate all the numbers on your credit card)*   EXPIRATION DATE

▢▢▢▢ ▢▢▢▢ ▢▢▢▢ ▢▢▢▢   ▢▢/▢▢

Day Phone ( )_____

SIGNATURE _____   DATE _____

NOTE: We ship best method available for your delivery address. Foreign orders are sent by air. Credit card or International M.O. only. For rush processing of your order, add an additional $10.00 per address. Available on money order & charge card orders only.

Errors and omissions excepted. Prices subject to change without notice.

ORDERING INFORMATION

Customer Service Questions? Please call us between 9:00am–11:00pm EST Monday to Friday at 1-800-899-5111. Local and foreign customers call 513-346-4160 for orders and customer service

100% One-Year Risk-Free Guarantee. If you are not completely satisfied with any product–for any reason, no matter how long after you received it–we'll be happy to give you a prompt exchange, credit, or refund, as you wish. Simply return your purchase to us, and please let us know why you were dissatisfied–it will help us to provide better products and services in the future. *Shipping and handling fees are non-refundable.*

Telephone Orders For faster service you may place your orders by calling Toll Free 24 hours a day, 7 days a week, 365 days per year. When you call, please have your credit card ready.

1·800·899·5111
24 HOURS A DAY
FAX YOUR ORDER (866) 280-7619

Complete and mail with full payment to: Dragon Door Publications, P.O. Box 1097, West Chester, OH 45071

Please print clearly
Sold To: A

Name_____

Street_____

City_____

State_____ Zip_____

Day phone*_____
* Important for clarifying questions on orders

Please print clearly
SHIP TO: *(Street address for delivery)* B

Name_____

Street_____

City_____

State_____ Zip_____

Email_____

Warning to foreign customers:
The Customs in your country may or may not tax or otherwise charge you an additional fee for goods you receive. Dragon Door Publications is charging you only for U.S. handling and international shipping. Dragon Door Publications is in no way responsible for any additional fees levied by Customs, the carrier or any other entity.

Item #	Qty.	Item Description	Item Price	A or B	Total

HANDLING AND SHIPPING CHARGES • NO COD'S
Total Amount of Order Add:

$00.00 to $24.99 add $5.00
$25.00 to $39.99 add $6.00
$40.00 to $59.99 add $7.00
$60.00 to $99.99

$100.00 to $129.99 add $12.00
$130.00 to $169.99 add $14.00
$170.00 to $199.99 add $16.00
$200.00 to $299.99 add $18.00
$300.00 and up add $20.00

Canada & Mexico add $8.00. All other countries triple U.S. charges.

Total of Goods	
Shipping Charges	
Rush Charges	
Kettlebell Shipping Charges	
OH residents add 6% sales tax	
MN residents add 6.5% sales tax	
Total Enclosed	

Method of Payment ❑ Check ❑ M.O. ❑ Mastercard ❑ Visa ❑ Discover ❑ Amex

Account No. *(Please indicate all the numbers on your credit card)*   EXPIRATION DATE

□□□□ □□□□ □□□□ □□□□   □□/□□

Day Phone (   )_____

SIGNATURE _____   DATE _____

NOTE: We ship best method available for your delivery address. Foreign orders are sent by air. Credit card or International M.O. only. For rush processing of your order, add an additional $10.00 per address. Available on money order & charge card orders only.

Errors and omissions excepted. Prices subject to change without notice.

DDP 03/04

ORDERING INFORMATION

Customer Service Questions? Please call us between 9:00am–11:00pm EST Monday to Friday at 1-800-899-5111. Local and foreign customers call 513-346-4160 for orders and customer service

100% One-Year Risk-Free Guarantee. If you are not completely satisfied with any product–for any reason, no matter how long after you received it–we'll be happy to give you a prompt exchange, credit, or refund, as you wish. Simply return your purchase to us, and please let us know why you were dissatisfied–it will help us to provide better products and services in the future. *Shipping and handling fees are non-refundable.*

Telephone Orders For faster service you may place your orders by calling Toll Free 24 hours a day, 7 days a week, 365 days per year. When you call, please have your credit card ready.

1·800·899·5111
24 HOURS A DAY
FAX YOUR ORDER (866) 280-7619

Complete and mail with full payment to: Dragon Door Publications, P.O. Box 1097, West Chester, OH 45071

Please print clearly

Sold To: **A**

Name_____

Street_____

City_____

State_____ Zip _____

Day phone*_____
* Important for clarifying questions on orders

Please print clearly

SHIP TO: *(Street address for delivery)*   **B**

Name_____

Street_____

City_____

State_____ Zip _____

Email_____

Warning to foreign customers:
The Customs in your country may or may not tax or otherwise charge you an additional fee for goods you receive. Dragon Door Publications is charging you only for U.S. handling and international shipping. Dragon Door Publications is in no way responsible for any additional fees levied by Customs, the carrier or any other entity.

ITEM #	QTY.	ITEM DESCRIPTION	ITEM PRICE	A OR B	TOTAL

HANDLING AND SHIPPING CHARGES • NO COD'S
Total Amount of Order Add:

$00.00 to $24.99 add $5.00	$100.00 to $129.99 add $12.00	
$25.00 to $39.99 add $6.00	$130.00 to $169.99 add $14.00	
$40.00 to $59.99 add $7.00	$170.00 to $199.99 add $16.00	
$60.00 to $99.99	$200.00 to $299.99 add $18.00	
	$300.00 and up add $20.00	

Canada & Mexico add $8.00. All other countries triple U.S. charges.

Total of Goods	
Shipping Charges	
Rush Charges	
Kettlebell Shipping Charges	
OH residents add 6% sales tax	
MN residents add 6.5% sales tax	
TOTAL ENCLOSED	

METHOD OF PAYMENT ❏ CHECK ❏ M.O. ❏ MASTERCARD ❏ VISA ❏ DISCOVER ❏ AMEX

Account No. *(Please indicate all the numbers on your credit card)*   EXPIRATION DATE

▢▢▢▢ ▢▢▢▢ ▢▢▢▢ ▢▢▢▢   ▢▢/▢▢

Day Phone (   )_____

SIGNATURE _____   DATE _____

NOTE: We ship best method available for your delivery address. Foreign orders are sent by air. Credit card or International M.O. only. For rush processing of your order, add an additional $10.00 per address. Available on money order & charge card orders only.

Errors and omissions excepted. Prices subject to change without notice.

DDP 03/04